Cheri
Barren Plains

A Woman's Journey from Mental Illness to a Prison Cell

Larry L Franklin

chipmunkapublishing
the mental health publisher

Larry L Franklin

All rights reserved, no part of this publication may be reproduced by any means, electronic, mechanical photocopying, documentary, film or in any other format without prior written permission of the publisher.

> Published by
> Chipmunkapublishing
> PO Box 6872
> Brentwood
> Essex CM13 1ZT
> United Kingdom

http://www.chipmunkapublishing.com

Copyright © Larry L Franklin 2010

Chipmunkapublishing gratefully acknowledge the support of Arts Council England.

Cherry Blossoms & Barren Plains

For Dani and Rebecca Bivens, and all victims of preventable tragedies

Larry L Franklin

Cherry Blossoms & Barren Plains

Contents

Acknowledgments
Author's Note
Prologue: Fall Day, 2004

Part One

1. Paper Trail to Madness
2. "I take my meds and no one hurts me anymore"
3. Second Chance
4. "In a little white house down by the river"
5. "I just needed more help"
6. Greek Tragedies
7. Little White Box
8. Broken Mind
9. Confession
10. LaSalle County Jail
11. Crazy or Not

Part Two

12. Fish Heads in an Open Bag
13. Preventable Tragedies
14. "From the city streets, to the county jail"
15. "Treatment works, if you can get it"

16. "No need for a prison cell"

Epilogue: Winter Day, 2009

Cherry Blossoms & Barren Plains

Acknowledgements

I gratefully acknowledge Jason Pegler, the CEO at Chipmunka Publishing Company, for choosing to publish my work. I thank the staff at Chipmunka for their assistance.

I particularly thank my editor, Diana Hume George, for her support and guidance through the completion of my manuscript. My appreciation goes to research psychologist Charles Meliska for reading my work, and correcting me when I reached flawed conclusions. His intellect and sensitivity were much needed attributes as I dealt with the complexities of mental illness. And to professional psychotherapist Janet Coffman, for teaching me the intricacies and power of psychotherapy.

My love and affection go to my wife, Paula, for her support and understanding when my mind was busy processing Becca's story. My work demanded such an emotional cost that I was left empty, waiting for my soul to recharge.

Kudos to Mackenzie Wicoff for her stunning artwork.

Special thanks go to Becca for granting me entrance into her deepest thoughts. Her cooperation and determination to delve into the mysteries of her mental illness were essential in telling her story. It is my hope and prayer that my efforts bring Becca a new-found peace, and that her children will have a better understanding of their mother's life.

Larry L Franklin

Cherry Blossoms & Barren Plains

Author Biography

Larry L. Franklin is 66 years old and resides in Makanda, Illinois. Franklin holds Bachelor's and Master's degrees in Music, and performed in the U.S. Navy Band, located in Washington, D. C., from 1976 to 1971. From 1972 through 1975, Larry taught music at Southern Illinois University. In 1976, he completed requirements for a Certified Financial Planner designation and maintained a successful investment business until 2007, when he retired to devote his energies to writing. In 2003, Larry received an MFA in Creative Non-Fiction from Goucher College in Baltimore, Maryland.

Each professional pursuit left Franklin with an unsatisfying emptiness that pushed him into marathon running, where he pounded the country roads longing for an answer just around the bend. Then, in 1998, and without warning, repressed memories broke through his subconscious mind like a runaway train, and left him afraid to leave his home. He was diagnosed with Post Traumatic Stress Disorder (PTSD) with dissociative features. What followed were years of psychotherapy where he explored a physically and sexually abusive childhood. Now his problems have been reduced to a persistent mild depression which is controlled by medication and talk therapy. The therapeutic process unleashed his creative side, a new-found ability to write, and an unquenchable curiosity about the human mind. Larry now devotes his time writing about the mentally ill and victims of injustice who yearn for a voice to tell their story.

Larry L Franklin

Cherry Blossoms & Barren Plains

Author's Note

This is a work of nonfiction. Except where indicated, all names are real. Some thirty interviews with Rebecca Bivens were held at the Dwight Correctional Center in Dwight, Illinois, and on all occasions, each lasted four hours. Since the use of paper, pencils, and recording devices was prohibited, all conversations were recalled and transcribed from memory and later proofread by Rebecca to ensure accuracy. Telephone calls and letters were exchanged between Rebecca and myself. Medical records and trial transcripts, and interviews with psychologists and other mental health practitioners provided detailed information as well. In addition, countless articles and books about mental illness, prison life, violence against women, and my personal experience as an abuse victim helped explain why Rebecca made her journey from mental illness to a prison cell.

Larry L Franklin

Cherry Blossoms & Barren Plains

Prologue:
Fall Day, 2004

This was the place where I first heard about Cherry Blossoms and Barren Plains. A tall, chain-link fence, topped with rows of razor wire, circled the building that turned a rich, rust color after a steady rain or a wet winter snow, and suddenly lightened like sand when warmed by the morning sun. This stone-walled castle-like structure just off Interstate 55, one mile west of Dwight, Illinois, and seventy-five miles south of Chicago, was home for 1,039 women. Opened in November 24, 1930 as the Oakdale Reformatory for Women, it was subsequently renamed the Illinois State Reformatory for Women and finally the Dwight Correctional Center in 1973.

This was where I first met Rebecca Bivens. Her hair had darkened to a reddish-brown with an occasional streak of gray, her five-foot ten-inch stature made you take a second look, and her eyes, the purest blue you can imagine, mirrored sadness. We sat in dark plastic chairs that bent slightly with a shift in weight and we leaned forward onto a small circular table that wobbled on the uneven floor. This place – a room with twenty-foot ceilings, concrete walls and tiled floors, and vending machines that lined the outer walls like toy soldiers – was called the visit room, the place where visitors and inmates talked and sometimes shared secrets.

I was writing a book about Rita Nitz, who, like Rebecca, was an inmate at the Dwight Correctional Center. Rita was convicted of first-degree murder and sentenced to life without parole, not for participating in the murder but for watching her abusive husband beat a man with a baseball bat. I had asked for the names of other inmates who would broaden my insight into women's prisons. It was Rita who gave me Rebecca's name. Except for the scant details I had obtained on the Illinois Department of Correction's website – Rebecca was convicted of first-degree murder and sentenced to life in prison – I knew little more. Inmates keep their sordid pasts close to the vest, knowing that any openness leaves them more vulnerable to their fellow prisoners.

After three years of conversations with Rita, reading books on the incarceration of women, and my imagined visions of a 6 x 9 foot cell, my mind had created a rigid picture of life at Dwight. Two metal beds and a steel sink were bolted to the wall, and an exposed toilet gripped the floor. Privacy was a distant memory. With little room to turn, one inmate's exhale became the other inmate's inhale, and the stale air held a slight smell of body fluids and human skin. Friendships were discouraged as inmates were continually moved to different cells, reminding me of musical chairs – the game children play.

On this day, the visit room was filled with the typical visitors: an inmate sat with a church volunteer here to spread the word of God, an older couple waited to see their daughter, a grandmother brought a child to see her mother, a man waited to see his wife, and someone like myself listened for a story. This was the inmates' living room, where they entertained company and longed to be loved.

I suppose it was all of the pain and suffering that I had witnessed at Dwight. That must have been why I was so surprised when Rebecca said, "Prison is the best place I've ever been. I take my meds everyday and no one hurts me anymore." I was momentarily stunned while I gathered my thoughts.

"What do you mean, this is the best place you've ever been?"

"If it hadn't been for prison, I'd be dead," Rebecca said. Prior to prison, she was psychotic and heard imaginary voices. While her husband inflicted pain and the doctors prescribed medication, Rebecca had times when she didn't remember when one day gave into the next.

"Go ahead and ask me anything," she offered. "I have nothing to hide. I killed my five-year-old stepdaughter, but I don't remember doing it. I loved her so much and I think about her every day." Rebecca was found guilty but mentally ill, and was sentenced to life without parole.

I couldn't help but ask, "If you don't remember doing it, how do you know that you killed your stepdaughter?"

"Because they told me that I did," she answered.

It was here, in a prison for women, where Rebecca praised the beauty of Cherry Blossoms in Spring, and then blasted the starkness of Barren Plains; an image of emotional highs that shifted to the lowest of lows, and back again; a manic state so grandiose that she wanted nothing less, followed by a depression that drove her yearning to end it all. Mental health practitioners call this bipolar disorder, sometimes referred to as manic-depressive illness, which currently affects some 2.5 million American adults. Rebecca calls this her world of Cherry Blossoms and Barren Plains.

Rebecca described her state of mind when first incarcerated at the Dwight Correctional Center. "I spent six months in the mental wing," she said. "It was so scary. I mean the screaming and yelling made my skin crawl." She talked of other inmates, mostly young women who had dropped into madness. Some made it out, while others were not safe to be in a normal prison environment. Through an enforced medication regime and weekly psychotherapy, Rebecca demonstrated enough improvement to be transferred to the general population.

Despite the gains, the violent men in her life had left an enduring mark. Each time she came face to face with a male guard, her fears came home. "Just the sight of a man freaked me out." She cried and screamed and slipped into a panic, followed by a stint in a segregated cell until the tears passed and the image of a man faded.

"What about the female guards?" I asked. "Did you have a problem with them?"

"No," Becca answered. "It was only when a man approached me. But now things are different. A male guard can walk my way and yell at me and I can throw it right back. It doesn't bother me. Now I'm taking my meds and no one is hurting me."

Still, Rebecca would rather be in a mental hospital where she would receive therapy and come to understand what she had done. Six slow years after the death of her five-year-old step daughter, Becca doesn't remember what happened. "Dani was her name. She was like my own daughter and I loved her a lot. There's not a day that goes by without me thinking of her or wondering what I did. A psychiatrist said I might remember it some day. But right now, I don't remember a thing."

Rebecca's revelations hit me hard. I knew how missing chunks of memory can sink into the deepest part of your brain; sometimes never recovered, other times appearing when you least expect. Psychiatrists call them repressed memories that are meant to protect you from traumatic experiences that are too difficult for your brain to process. Mine were buried for decades until they broke through like a run-away train and left me afraid to leave my home. I was diagnosed with Post Traumatic Stress Disorder (PTSD) with dissociative features. PTSD is an anxiety disorder that can develop after exposure to one, or a series of traumatic events in which grave physical harm occurred or was threatened. Dissociative features refers to an inability to recall important personal information, usually of traumatic nature. What followed were years of psychotherapy where I explored an abusive childhood, and, in the process, developed an unquenchable curiosity about the human mind. Now my problems have been reduced to a persistent mild depression. Medication and talk therapy keep the big bear away.

I was struck by the mental illness that had pushed Rebecca to kill someone she truly loved. It reminded me of other people gone mad, who went on killing sprees, or squeezed the life from their children. Those were the kinds of stories that made me wonder why. We have read about them in the morning newspaper, or heard stories on the evening news, and then we worried and stewed until our coffee turned cold. But this was the first time I had come face to face with someone who had taken a child's life. Any uneasiness on my part was quickly overcome by my curiosity, and a sense of commonality that I felt with Rebecca. We shared a desire to understand what caused her mental illness, the role that domestic violence played in her downward spiral, the confused maze of mental health services, and why society tends to look the other way. Looking back, though, I believe that Rebecca had been waiting for a confidant to accompany her on the four-year journey that we were about to begin, and for some unspoken reason, I was the one.

In time, I obtained a large portion of her mental health records. Psychiatrists from different treatment centers had diagnosed her with bipolar disorder, a secondary diagnosis of acute borderline personality disorder, and post-traumatic stress disorder. When I had the proof of Rebecca's mental illness, we began a story that became much larger than her own. It is a narrative of mental illness with all of its ramifications: the biological and environmental causes; the treatment of mental illness from the nineteenth to the twenty-first century; the lack of society's understanding of a disease that plagues millions of people each day, and challenges our national budget; and the residual effects on family and friends ill-equipped to handle the demands of someone who suffers from a severe mental illness. Rebecca's illness was aggravated by the violent men in her life, which was another story looking to be told. Like so many battered women, she preferred a fist to her face, a stab from a knife, and a couple of broken ribs to the thought of living alone. Her illness, together with a violent environment, was a pattern as predictable as the quiet before a storm.

Those who struggle with a severe mental illness, or a friend or family member who deals with a loved one gone mad, may find solace in the fact that you are not alone. Such illness is as real as a cancerous brain tumor, and deserves the compassion of a society that too often looks the other way. For those who have never felt the ultimate highs twist and turn into fits of rage, and then plunge into a depression so bad that you beg for a way to die, this is a story that you must read.

There was never any hesitation from Rebecca or myself that her story had to be told. Usually I think long and hard before I make what could become a three to four year commitment. But this time there was no choice. This was a calling. We began a series of four-hour visits, some thirty in all, in the visit room at the Dwight Correctional Center. Amidst tables of inmates and visitors, and the smell of popcorn in the air, we leaned across that same small table that wobbled on the uneven floor. That's where her story began to unfold.

Larry L Franklin

Cherry Blossoms & Barren Plains

Part One

Larry L Franklin

Cherry Blossoms & Barren Plains

Paper Trail to Madness

The town, dissected by the Fox and Illinois rivers, was surrounded by fields of wheat, corn stalks that reached heights of eight feet, and beans so thick that you could walk across the field and your feet would never touch the ground. Ottawa, a farming community of some 18,000 residents, shared the same old-fashioned look – streets lined with white-framed houses marked by patches of brick – as those found in neighboring communities of Midwestern Illinois. While a plainness accompanied the flat farmland, the rich black top-soil, outdoor water sports, and a hospital that employed six hundred employees made Ottawa a good place to live.

On January 24, 1993, Rebecca Muller, a fair-skinned 26-year-old mother of four, with long hair the redness of Illinois rhubarb, told her story to Dojna Barr, M.D., the admitting physician at the Community Hospital of Ottawa (CHO). Just months earlier, Becca, as she was called, went to work but didn't come home. She left her family and escaped to a neighboring community where she found an apartment in a worn-down building and waited tables at a local bar. Her whereabouts were unknown. When her mania turned to depression, she called her parents for help, and when she agreed to check into a mental hospital, they brought her home.

Becca spoke of troubled times and a troubled marriage, as Barr scribbled her words onto the admission summary. The patient overdosed on Tylenol in September 1992 and continues to have suicidal thoughts accompanied by fatigue, severe sleep disturbance, racing thoughts, uncontrollable rage, headaches, poor concentration and comprehension, decreased sexual desire, excessive guilt about her children, and an urge to run and leave her family. While a weak coping system makes it impossible for her to explore a past rape, the borderline disorder interferes with any therapeutic relationship, giving rise to feelings of rage and anger, and thoughts against the therapist.

Barr's principal diagnosis of bipolar disorder, mixed, was followed by a secondary diagnosis of acute borderline personality disorder, and a history of rape with post-traumatic stress syndrome. Severe mood swings and suicidal thoughts required that Becca be stabilized beyond the phase of a comprehensive work-up. A one week stay in the Community Hospital of Ottawa was the beginning of a paper trail documenting a history of mental illness that led to an unimaginable conclusion on November 23, 1998: the day when Becca killed her five-year-old step daughter.

It was as if someone or something, possibly alien, took over her mind. I can see how an imaginary octopus-like creature might have controlled her thoughts. Living in the lowest part of her brain and hidden by darkness, this creature, the one I imagined, reached outward with its eight tentacles, each lined with two rows of suction cups, and latched onto family members and friends and strangled them hard. No one escaped its grip. When threatened, it released an inky-black liquid that allowed it to slip away. Even if one of its tentacles was severed, one quickly regrew, making it impossible to kill.

This octopus-like creature, the one that I imagined, the one that invaded Becca's mind, is called bipolar disorder, also known as manic-depressive illness. More than 2.5 million American adults, or roughly one percent of the population, struggle with bipolar disorder. This disease manifests itself as abnormalities in brain chemistry and in the structure and/or activity of certain brain circuits, causing extreme swings in moods, energy and functioning. Kay Redfield Jamison, author of *An Unquiet Mind*, says; "Manic-depression distorts moods and thoughts, incites dreadful behaviors, destroys the basis of rational thought, and too often erodes the desire and will to live." Jamison, a psychiatrist, and herself a victim of bipolar disorder, sees the illness as "biological in its origins, yet one that feels psychological in the experience..."

Becca's bipolar disorder was "mixed," meaning that her symptoms of mania and depression – the highs and lows – were experienced at the same time, bouncing quickly, like a rubber ball on a wooden floor. The addictive feelings of pleasure could instantaneously switch to rage, leaving her to lash out at whoever was near. At times, her mood swings were accompanied by psychotic symptoms: hallucinations and also delusions, those false beliefs not subject to reason. The psychotic symptoms magnified her moods, causing the mania to be more grandiose and the depression to be more unspeakable.

Barr gave a secondary diagnosis of borderline personality disorder(BPD). According to the National Institute of Mental Health (NIMH), roughly two per cent of adults, mostly young women, have BPD – an illness "characterized by pervasive instability in mood, inter-personal relationships, self-image, and behavior." People with BPD are more likely to be victims of violence; forty to seventy-one percent of patients with BPD have been sexually abused by non-caregivers; and some twenty percent of psychiatric hospitalizations are patients afflicted with BPD. As with bipolar disorder, most studies suggest a change in the brain chemistry and in the structure and/or activity of certain brain circuits as contributing to the development of BPD. Together, bipolar and borderline personality disorders create a current of mood swings, irritability, and aggression that only the strongest can survive.

Except for the construction underway, Becca doesn't remember anything unusual or striking about the Community Hospital of Ottawa. "It was like any hospital," she later said. The building, a concrete structure with massive windows, looked modern; the fourth floor served drug rehabilitation and mental health; and Becca's room had four hospital beds filled with like women searching for simple answers. Beth, an 18-year-old, had cut and mutilated her young body as she studied the sight of oozing blood. Joanne had ingested large amounts of drugs and alcohol, hoping to cope with her abusive husband. And then there was Mary Jean, the woman of many lives, who heard voices and changed identities and seemed to bounce off the walls, never reaching a resting place. In just a few days, the four of them became friends as they shared the commonality of mental illness. "We leaned on each other," Becca said.

Becca described each day as structured with activities that fit together like a jigsaw puzzle. *We showered at 6:00 a.m., ate breakfast at 7:00, and had group therapy at 8:00 a.m. when we received our morning meds. Two hours later, we ate lunch and had time to ourselves. Then we walked the grounds for an hour and a half. That's when we grew close. From 3:00 to 5:00 p.m. was television followed by dinner, 5:00 to 8:00 p.m. was visitation, 8:00 to 9:00 p.m. was another group session followed by more meds followed by snacks at 9:00 and bed by 11:00 p.m. On Tuesdays and Thursdays we went bowling, on Friday nights our families gave us money to buy pizza and rent movies. We were allowed to stay up until midnight. During groups we worked hard on ourselves. There was a lot of anger and sadness. They tried to teach us coping skills to deal with the people who made our lives unbearable. Sometimes we had family groups which usually turned into a screaming match. In case we needed to have our meds changed, we saw the psychiatrist twice a week I think I would have done better if they would have left me at CHO. I've always wanted to deal with my problems, and wanted to know why I was so messed up. I wanted to get better.*

One week after her admission to CHO, Barr wrote the hospital's course of action on Becca's discharge form. Lithium was started at 400 mg in slow release form at bedtime; 75 mg of Wellbutrin, one every second day in the first week and then one daily; and 1 mg of Klonopin at bedtime. While Lithium was intended to treat the manic state of the bipolar illness, Wellbutrin was to reduce depression, and Clonopin was intended to reduce anxiety. Barr suggested that therapy needed to be more supportive, with a cognitive approach, and that when Becca improved, she needed to learn better coping mechanisms and to slowly explore the past rape. Becca was still vulnerable when dealing with intimacy and other marital problems. The husband, according to Barr, didn't participate in a social history or talk with the physicians at CHO. Since Becca was believed to be integrated without any suicidal or homicidal thoughts, she was referred to her previous therapist and family physician. Becca was discharged on February 1, 1993, to her mother.

Two months later, death cheated her again. Becca swallowed a fistful of Lithium pills. She had struggled with fatigue and a lifeless mood as she fought the new medications being funneled into her brain. She slept often, waiting for her mind to adjust to chemicals promised to soften her moods and make her sane. At the same time, Becca continued seeing her psychologist, Truty Kirchaffer, on a weekly basis – sometimes with her mother, Carolyn, and sometimes with her husband, Larry. On one such visit, the three of them, Larry, Carolyn, and Becca – each with a short fuse that could be ignited by the slightest irritant – sat in Kirchaffer's office. Tension filled the air. The four children and Carolyn's friend sat in the waiting room. While Larry and Carolyn blamed each other for a share of Becca's pain, Becca wondered why she was broken. "I can't remember what my mother said to Larry," Becca later said. "I just remember that he was pissed off and stormed out of the room. My mother took me and the kids to our house that night. I thought Larry went out drinking somewhere. He did that sometimes when he got mad."

"It must have been around 11:00 p.m.," Becca remembered. Three of the children were sleeping while Becca and Alyssa, the youngest of the four children, were playing on the bed – cooing and laughing like most babies and mothers do. But in Becca's world, playful moments were often mere preludes to violence. There was the sound of a lock and the opening of a door. Becca turned to look, while Alyssa watched her daddy walk into the room. "He was searching through the closet," Becca later recalled. "I thought he wanted a suitcase. Maybe he was going to leave for the night." But the steel-gray object, about the size of a baby doll, that he pulled from the closet was partially hidden by his hanging shirt. He left the room. Minutes later, Larry, a broad-shouldered, stout man standing five-feet ten inches and carrying some 200 to 210 pounds, returned with a fully-loaded gun. His black hair was thick and his mustache was full and a small metal ring hung from his left ear. His brown eyes peered through the thick lenses of his wire-rimmed glasses. He pressed the gun muzzle hard and tight against her face. "Go ahead and kill me," Becca said, holding Alyssa to her side. "Let's get this over with." Click. The sound of metal striking metal was followed by a brief silence when Becca and Larry knew the gun had not fired. As Larry left the room, Becca called Carolyn to tell her how she was nearly killed. But her words were cut short when Larry returned and ripped the telephone from the wall. The house came alive with the sound of screaming children running with their mother to a corner of the house. Minutes later, three policemen responded to Carolyn's plea for help and broke down the door and pushed Larry's face to the floor.

After stripping Larry of all his guns, a policeman asked Becca if she wanted to stay or be taken to a safe place. Becca, like most battered women, chose to stay. But when Larry said that he had plenty of knives, the policemen took Becca and the children to Carolyn's house. One policeman told Becca that she was lucky. "Your husband was so drunk that he loaded the gun improperly. That's why it didn't fire."

In the days that followed, Becca and the children stayed with her mother before moving back with Larry. Depression moved Becca to a lonely place where death was her companion. Perhaps death sang words of seduction and eternal peace; a misty, cloud-like song for a lover. Hidden in the darkness of her bedroom, Becca swallowed fifty Lithium capsules. Minutes later, Larry found her lifeless body stretched out across the floor; perhaps her eyelids were half closed and her eyes were still. Larry rushed her rag-like body to the St. James emergency room, where death was denied when a tireless physician pumped her stomach dry.

Two weeks later, on April 15, 1993, Kirchaffer asked the

physicians at CHO to follow Becca for medication. As before, Becca repeated her story of troubled times and a failed marriage, while Archibald Hutchinson, M.D., the admitting physician at CHO, transferred his thoughts to the admission form.

The patient, a 26-year-old mother of four, is on Lithium Carbonate 300 mg by mouth, three times per day, as well as Wellbutrin 75 mg in the morning. She is being harassed by her husband and her mother who are in collusion to keep the couple together. The patient's anxiety level has increased and she has racing thoughts, confusion, poor concentration, high distractibility, feelings of worthlessness and hopelessness and overwhelming guilt about her children. She feels more depressed than her last hospitalization and has prominent suicidal thoughts. Except when having rage attacks, the patient admits to feeling fatigued. Her mood swings from baseline to depression or severe irritability, and her anger lacks control, as when she trashed her home prior to the failed suicide. Patient admits to feeling easily hurt by criticism from others, unable to make important decisions and agrees with others even though she believes they are wrong. Patient admits to sexual abuse while she was a child. The family history has two cousins with a history of depression. Patient's first marriage, which lasted just nine months, was to a violent man who was the father of her first child. Impulse control is markedly impaired as noted by suicidal gesture and uncontrollable rage attacks; insight and judgment are markedly impaired. The patient is placed on suicidal and local precaution, and prescribed Lithium Carbonate 300 mg three times per day as well as Wellbutrin 75 mg in the morning. Corgard, a beta blocker for impulse control and a different serotonin re-uptake inhibitor are being considered.

For Becca, life at CHO was good. It was a retreat from her violent world that rotated and spun in a universe inhabited by strangers who misunderstood her. But in the safety of a hospital, no one held a gun to her head or belittled her for a broken life. It was a place where the psychiatrists tweaked her medication and taught her some coping skills, where patients shared their sameness and wondered why society called them insane. This stay lasted for a month, giving her time for stronger bonds with other patients who shared her complicated thoughts. They talked and listened and sometimes disagreed, like family members circling the table after an evening meal.

They called him Jason, this 42-year-old man at CHO. He was

Cherry Blossoms & Barren Plains

like a bird with a broken wing; they said he would never fly. He was a genius; that's what his parents said. "He was going to be a doctor and had to be perfect and had a nervous breakdown," Becca added. "He was schizo." Like so many, Jason didn't take his medication and never seemed to improve. He shunned closeness and cut himself to let the demons out. But one day, while walking down the hallway, he stopped and looked into Becca's eyes. "Pretty blue," he said. Then things began to change.

"He started taking his meds and began to eat," Becca said. "He listened to whatever I said. He wouldn't let me get physically close to him but we started to play games. His favorite was 1500 Rummy. It was a good feeling. His parents even offered me a job to help take care of Jason. But I said no. My kids were still little and I was afraid of getting attached to him."

Becca improved at CHO, showing a gentler side that was smothered in her outside world. Even hospital employees told Becca that when she recovered, she might consider working with the mentally ill. "They said I had a way with them," Becca smiled. It was evident when she talked with Joey, an oversized teenage boy who had Down's Syndrome. His anger broke through as he struck whoever was in his way. In time, Becca taught him to look into her eyes, to count to ten, and feel the anger move away. She remembers hearing Joey stop and count to ten.

The routine was the same as before – a highly structured schedule where time had a purpose. There were the group sessions, the daily distributions of medications, the planned meals, a bi-weekly check-in with the psychiatrists, and the daily walks. This time, Becca shared a semi-private room with Joanne, the woman she met during her earlier stay, the one who took large amounts of drugs and alcohol to ease memories of an abusive husband. "We were roommates and talked about a lot of stuff," Becca said. "We tried to figure out our lives." They remained friends on the outside, until Larry convinced Becca that Joanne was taking advantage of her, just using Becca to baby-sit her children.

Becca said that most of the patients at CHO were there for short periods of time, not long enough to form lasting relationships. She remembered an 18-year-old girl, Sarah might have been her name, who sliced her wrists and wanted to die. "They sent her to Zellers, the state hospital in Peoria," Becca recalled. "I felt so bad and scared for her. She was too young to go to a place like that. There were some really sick people, but to be so young and want to die. It broke my heart. If only I could have gotten her to open up. She was full of silent cries."

Even in CHO, life was not always safe. Dan was placed at CHO rather than in jail where he most likely belonged. Medium-built and some five-feet ten-inches tall, Dan was a violent man, who later began serving a forty-five year sentence for murder. His slick black hair was short on top and grew down his neck, and his mustache turned up at the corners. Tattoos reached from his wrists to his biceps. At first he stared at Becca, followed by the occasional "Hi," and finally, the sleazy remarks; "Would you like to see the tattoo of a horse on my penis?" Becca turned and walked away, trying to maintain a safe distance from this man. At the time, Becca was placed on Trazadone, an anti-depressant sometimes used as a sleep aid; one common side effect was extreme drowsiness and an urge to sleep. "The drug knocked me out," Becca said. "It made me feel like I was half in and half out." One night at CHO, while most patients slept, Becca awoke when Dan rammed his tattooed penis down her throat. "I couldn't breathe," she said. "I wanted to scream, but I couldn't. I was going back and forth between being conscious and unconscious. The next time I woke up, he was on top of me." Becca believes that the staff heard her struggle. When they yelled at Dan, he stopped.

On the following day, according to Becca, the hospital staff wanted her to press charges against Dan. But Becca said she didn't know if it really happened. She was pumped full of mind-altering drugs that plays with reality. Maybe it was a dream, or maybe she didn't want Larry or her mother to know. So the hospital promised not to tell anyone and she promised as well.

Becca was discharged from CHO on May 20, 1993. The medication instructions at the time of discharge were to continue patient on Lithium Carbonate, 600 mg in the morning and at bed time; Corgard, 40 mg in the morning and at bed time; Zoloft, 100 mg in the morning and at bed time; Haldol, 5 mg at bedtime; and Artane, 2 mg at bedtime. Patient is to follow up with her psychologist and continue her after-care at CHO every Tuesday at 6:30 p.m. for medication management. Prognosis is guarded-to-poor, secondary to the patient's longstanding characterological problems.

Just six days later, on May 26, 1993, her feelings moved fast and furious, like a deflating balloon bouncing off paneled walls. When she threatened to cut her arms with a razor blade, Larry brought her to the emergency room. "I can't take it anymore," she said. "I'm going crazy." While Archibald Hutchinson, another physician at CHO, listened and watched Becca shift her weight from one foot to the other, he recorded a familiar story. Patient has a history of very labile – fluctuating/changing rapidly – mood, has carried a diagnosis of bipolar disorder, mixed, as well as borderline personality disorder. Patient believes that her husband and her mother are in collusion, which sets her off in rage attacks when she becomes aggressive. The patient admitted to racing thoughts, confusion, poor concentration, high distractibility, feelings of worthlessness, hopelessness and overwhelming guilt about her children as well as prominent suicidal thoughts. She complained more of anxiety than of depressive thoughts. The patient admitted to auditory hallucinations of various men telling her to hurt herself. She also complained of boredom, inability to control her rage, impulses, switching from baseline mood to depression, difficulty in interpersonal relationships as well as engaging in potentially self harming projects and decisions such as self-mutilation. Lithium Carbonate was started at 300 mg capsules, 2 capsules in the morning and in the evening; Inderal 20 mg, 1 tablet by mouth 2x per day; Tranxene 3.75 mg, 1 tablet by mouth, 3x per day. When in a controlled environment, the patient is less anxious, sleeps better, and feels less depressed.

Six more days passed when the physicians discharged Becca on an outpatient basis. While a careful aftercare plan was created, Becca's prognosis was poor. Her longstanding problems and poor coping skills offered little hope. But she was not a threat to hurt herself or others, leaving the physicians with no choice but to let her go.

Now, as we sat in the visit room at the Dwight Correctional Center, some twelve years after she was attacked by the man called Dan, she talked about her multiple stays at CHO. While some of the memories were muffled, others held the crisp chill of a morning frost. Becca recalled the dark times when she left CHO, the times when she wrestled her nightmares. "I couldn't remember what they were about," she recalled. "I just remember seeing knives, blood, lots of blood, and a tattoo."

"I take my meds and no one hurts me anymore."

It was early October 2005 and the air still held the warmness of a hot summer day. South of the Dwight Correctional Center, on highway 17 and three miles from the nearest town, tractors pulled farm machinery past the prison walls. To the east, cars traveled down Interstate 55. As inmates walked from one building to the next or mowed the prison lawn, they looked at passing cars that might take them to the nearest shopping mall, the local movie house, or perhaps a coffee shop to visit a friend. They longed for freedoms that were beyond their grasp. Just down the road was Steel's, a worn-down truck stop, where truckers sat on stools that lined a long counter top. They ate breakfast and drank black coffee and took deep pulls from their cigarettes. Red vinyl booths hugged the walls and large round tables marked the floor. A separate room was the hangout for local residents and farmers on a rainy day, and people like me, waiting to visit an inmate at Dwight's.

Inside the prison, the two of us, Becca and I, sat in dark-colored plastic chairs around a small circular table in the visit room. Four or five tables were filled with visitors and inmates; women dressed in yellow jump suits waited to be transferred to a prison in Lincoln, Illinois; and one inmate sat behind a glass wall where chains tied her to a metal stool.

Although I had received Becca's mental health records from the Community Hospital of Ottawa where she was a frequent patient from 1993 through 1994, the records were not obtained without some struggle. First, I secured a release form signed by Becca, which I sent to the hospital, which was then forwarded to their attorney. Months later, the attorney requested another release form signed by Becca and notarized by a prison official. Then, and only then, would the medical records be sent to Becca. And even after Becca's prompt response, the records were slow to follow.

One of Becca's family members sent an anonymous note to me suggesting that "Becca beat that poor little girl to death and is right where she belongs... And for me to make my money on someone else." Her mother said that like many times before, Becca was thinking only of herself, while other family members told her not to bring up the past. But we were committed, both Becca and I, to tell her story and let the public know what led to that terrible morning on November 23, 1998, when Becca killed her five-year-old step

Cherry Blossoms & Barren Plains

daughter.

We had met three or four times and exchanged letters, and she called me on Monday nights. For us, talk was easy. While each visit focused on Becca's story, I gave her a glimpse into my abusive childhood, when my brother took me to the barn. He was 13 and I was barely 7. It was that old red barn, just east of the machine shed and north of our two-story white house, where he had his way. Becca and I shared a common bond when people, who should have loved us, brought us hell. It was a feeling more easily felt than explained. And when her family asked about me, Becca said; "Well, he's not in prison, but we're pretty much the same."

At times, when Becca's mind seemed to drift, she shared the same quiet ways of her father, Brenton Reed, a six-foot five-inch, two-hundred-and-twenty pound man, with gray eyes and grayish-brown hair. "He had a good sense of humor," Becca said. "But some people thought he was a bit scary. I think that was because of his size." Perhaps his quiet ways were a reflection of his past, when his mind drifted back to his abusive father. "When my mom worked, me and my brother followed dad everywhere. To the store, maybe fishing, or just washing the clothes. He was a wonderful father." Becca believes that her mother, a heavy-set woman with short black hair and dark eyes, was the opposite of her father. "That's just how I saw her," Becca said. "Everything was her way or it was wrong. When something bad happened, she just wouldn't talk about it. You couldn't talk to her about sex, drugs, alcohol, or anything. I always thought that I was a disappointment to her." Becca hesitated, and then looked down. "She didn't tell me that she loved me until I was 31 years old. When I was in prison."

Today, the imagined voices are gone and the manic feelings are muffled by medications. She is a rational person, not unlike people on the outside, who struggle with the dull ache of a prolonged depression. Still, she has moments when the medications do not erase, but merely dampen her racing mind and the loneliness of despair. It's not unusual for Becca to leave the company of fellow inmates and seek the isolation of her cell. She continues to ask me for books of crossword puzzles to pacify a busy mind.

Becca's words, spoken during our first meeting, still interrupt my thoughts like a repeated refrain in a down-hearted song: "Prison is the best place I've ever been. I take my meds and no one hurts me anymore." Dr. Hutchinson saw it in 1994 when he said that Becca improved quickly in a controlled environment. The questions were obvious. If Becca, in 1994, when her prognosis was poor, had been placed in a mental hospital for extended care, would her future have been different? A retreat from her violent world might have provided proper monitoring of her medications; she might have developed better coping skills; and her step-daughter might still be alive. But without money, Becca could not afford the luxury of private care, and was left to societal whims.

***

I can only imagine how Becca's life might have been if she had lived during an earlier time. In France, during the late 18th and early 19th centuries, the therapeutic asylum, commonly called moral therapy, was born. It spread to the United States and migrated from the east cost to the Midwest and finally to the west coast. In Illinois, the movement, spearheaded by the physician Edward Mead, lawyer-politician William Thomas, and businessman Joseph O. King, became a state law on March 1, 1847 when Governor Augustus French signed the *Act to establish the Illinois State Hospital for the Insane*. Earlier, the mentally ill were placed in a county almshouse or poor house, as they were commonly called, where they were sometimes kept in cages or metal pens, sometimes naked or partially clothed. But the Act of 1847 entitled the mentally ill to the funding and care of the state. Supporters of the Act believed that a controlled environment provided a positive effect on the individual psychological process and thus altered behavior. In Joseph J. Mehr's book, *An Illustrated History of the Illinois Public Mental Health Services: 1847 to 2000*, he says, "the asylum movement of the 19th century was the state of the art approach of the time and in fact, was far better than what would have followed a century later."

In the fall of 1847, construction began on the first therapeutic asylum in Illinois. It followed the "Kirkbride Plan," named after Thomas Story Kirkbride, M.D., who, in 1840, was the Superintendent of the Pennsylvania Hospital for the Insane. The center section, reserved for offices and meeting rooms, was five stories built over a basement with an attic floor on top. To each side was a wing of three stories over a basement which served as a dormitory for patients: men in one wing, women in the other. Those patients who could pay had private rooms; the indigent, like Becca, lived in the dormitory. The asylum opened with an enrollment of 166 patients.

Cherry Blossoms & Barren Plains

If Becca had lived in Illinois during the mid 1800s, she would have been in a more tranquil setting where stress was reduced and kindness was ongoing; she would have been separated from the family and friends who sometimes wreaked anguish. After determining her level of insanity, a precise program of treatment would have been prescribed. Engage the mind and exercise the body; restore mental health and tranquilize the restless; and mitigate the sorrow of disease – these were the stated standards of the day.

In a typical day at a 19th century therapeutic asylum, Becca would have awakened at 4:45 a.m. in the summer and 5:15 a.m. in the winter. After making her bed, Becca would have received her medications. At 8:00 a.m., the physician would review Becca's progress and prescribe her activities for the day, and like other patients, she would have had a meaningful job – maybe physical labor, like working on a farm; maybe bookkeeping or working as a seamstress in a sewing shop. Noon was the main meal, followed by snacks at 4:00 p.m., and a light evening meal at 6:00 p.m. Organized games or exercise, religious services, and public meetings replaced idle time.

Although the asylum might appear like a spa or a plush resort, that was not the case. The asylum was filled with very disturbed patients whose minds served a different reality. And some treatments, like bloodletting, considered state of the art at the time, would seem medieval under today's standards. Physicians treated mania by bleeding the patient until they became lethargic and without emotion. According to Joseph Mehr, sedatives and narcotics were used to calm patients so that they could more easily accept counseling. Counter-irritants were used to stimulate the emotions. Emetics were used to induce vomiting and purgatives to cleanse the bowels.

The supporters of the therapeutic asylum believed that if the mental illness was caught soon enough and treated, the patient would likely be cured. It was an optimistic time when the combination of a controlled environment and proper treatment might have given a person like Becca a reason for hope.

***

Now, some one-hundred-and-fifty years later, while we sit in the visit room at the Dwight Correctional Center, we talk about many things. We talk about how her reality spun into madness; how she longs for answers about what happened in her life; and how the prison deals with her mental illness.

A report, *"Mental Health Treatment in State Prisons, 2000,"* compiled by the Bureau of Justice Statistics, stated that 9.9 percent of Illinois' 44,000 inmates that responded to their survey, were in counseling, and 6.7 percent were receiving psychotic medications. Among the state's 48 facilities, 31 provided counseling, 31 distributed psychotic medications, and 32 provided 24-hour mental health care.

"How does the prison deal with mental illness?" I asked.

"They say there's not enough counselors for us," she answered as her frustration grew. "I have to fight for every bit of help that I get."

"What do you mean?" I asked.

"We only get to see a psychiatrist once a month, if we're lucky. Sometimes our medicine runs out and we have to call over there and ask them to get us in as quick as possible. Sometimes we go for weeks without our medicine."

"When that happens, do you become anxious?" I asked.

"Yes. And when we get sick, they want to put you in a stripped cell and make you take your clothes off. No clothes, no mattress. You sleep on the concrete floor. You're only allowed finger foods. You can't use silverware." I couldn't help but visualize Becca curled up in a fetal position as she lay on the concrete floor. Perhaps the floor was drafty. Perhaps the silence was interrupted by the clang of a closing door or the groan of a nearby inmate. "Sometimes the staff makes fun of the girls when they are really sick. They agitate them on purpose just to see how they will act out. And then they call them nuts or crazy. It's really hard." Becca hesitated. "And when you're not feeling the greatest, you're just afraid to tell anyone. They'll just want to put you in the stripped cell and make you take all your clothes off."

Becca looked downward and seemed to focus on the table top. My mind wandered amidst the prison sounds: the sound of metal doors slamming shut; conversations concealed in whispered tones; and the homesick cries of a child watching her mother walk away. As bad as prison seemed, I was still reminded of that same downhearted song: "Prison is the best place I've ever been. I take my meds and no one hurts me anymore."

***

Cherry Blossoms & Barren Plains

It was another day in the visit room, a weekday when the visitors were few and our words hung stubbornly in the stale air. We were in the middle of our visit when she finished eating an ice cream sandwich. Her passion for the ice cream treat became our inside joke. She savored the snack like a wine connoisseur relishes a fine wine, and was known to polish off four sandwiches in a single visit. I joked with Becca that I had to take a second job to pay for all of the food I bought from the vending machines. She could go through $15 of snacks in a single visit. While working on the prison lawn, Becca had earned $15 per month, which she used at the commissary to buy writing paper, stamps, and a candy bar or two. But a recent shoulder injury had left her without work, and since she had begun to tell her story, her family refused to send her any money. The taste of chocolate or the occasional ice cream sandwich were just memories. (Now, some four years later, budget cuts have eliminated the monthly pay for assigned jobs. Any money to be used at the prison commissary must come from family or friends.)

I decided to ask the question I had asked so many times before. "Tell me about Al," I said. Al McAllister was Becca's first husband and Amanda's father.

"I don't like talking about him," she answered. "I don't want Amanda to get mad at me."

Since her twenty-one year-old Amanda had contact with her father, Becca was reluctant to say anything that might turn Amanda against her. "I understand," I said. "Still, it would help if I know something about him. Tell me, was he short or tall?"

Although reluctant, she began to talk. "He was around five feet eight inches and was a little heavy," she answered. Silence followed.

"Come on," I said. "You can tell me more than that. What was the color of his hair, his eyes? Tell me more."

"He had blond hair and blue eyes," she said in a disgusted tone.

"Did he have any distinguishing or special characteristics that attracted you to him?"

"There was nothing special about him," Becca shrugged.

"Well, did he have any marks on his face, tattoos? How about a mustache?"

"He had a mustache," she answered.

"Was it a big one, small one? What was it like?"

"It was just a mustache," she said, voice raising. "It was nothing special."

Each time I asked Becca to describe the men in her life, I frequently heard the description of an average man, of average height, average appearance, and average build. Everyone was average. Most of the men in her life seemed like an old pair of jeans that she slid into each day. Each pair was familiar, like the familiar feel of violent men. I remembered Becca telling me that she would rather have put up with the violence than being alone.

"When did you marry Al?"

"January 18, 1985. I was 18 and he was 23," Becca said. "I think I married him just to make my mom mad and to get out of the house. I don't think I ever loved him." She described the marriage as "okay" in the beginning, but it quickly deteriorated into a nightmare that lasted less than one year. Just months after the wedding, Becca was pregnant with Amanda and was to deliver the following November. She told me a series of stories that showed Al to be typical of the other men in her life.

A few months into their marriage, maybe in March or April, when Becca was pregnant with Amanda and was beginning to show, Becca and Al went to the local bar for an evening of dancing. Al saw an old girl friend and began kissing her on the dance floor. When Becca complained, he spit in Becca's face. Terry, a friend of Al's, offered to take Becca home. Al followed them to the parking lot, where he began punching Becca. When Terry intervened, the two of them got into a fight that didn't stop until the police arrived. Finally, Becca agreed to go home with Al, where he beat her, threw the telephone through the window, and trashed their trailer. Becca escaped to a nearby trailer and spent the night with their neighbor, who was the sister of Becca's Aunt Marlene.

"Al was a jealous man and hated anyone or anything that I loved. He kicked and hit my dog, Pork Chop. He said that I gave Pork Chop more attention than him. And then there was my kitten that he buried alive."

"What do you mean?" I asked in a surprised tone.

"I was at my mom and dad's," Becca said. "Aunt Marlene was at their house for a visit. Al called and said that I should come home. That he had buried my kitten alive. Me and Aunt Marlene raced back home and searched all over the place. We never found my kitten."

"Did he ever tell you where he buried the kitten?" I asked.

"No," she answered. "We never talked about it again."

She went on to say that their relationship continued to deteriorate until she couldn't stand his touch. "After we had sex, I'd go to the bathroom and throw up."

The fighting between Al and Becca continued. On one such night, some three months after the birth of Amanda, Al accused Becca of spending too much time with Amanda. "He said that Amanda was my life and that I didn't think about him," Becca said. "We were standing in the bedroom and I was holding Amanda. He grabbed Amanda and threw her onto the bed and she bounced and hit the wall. I picked up Amanda and her diaper bag and we left. I never went back and I filed for divorce."

In October, 1986, one month after she began seeing Larry, her divorce with Al was final. "Al stalked me and harassed me for months. Al and Larry were always getting into fights. Al stopped seeing Amanda and didn't spend any real time with her until she was about six years old. His parents made a point of seeing her, though."

"So you were married to four men? Al, Larry, Ciro and Chad. Is that right?

"Yes," she answered.

"Who was the father of your children?" I asked.

"Al was the father of Amanda. Larry was the father of my next three children. Then I had my tubes tied and that was it."

Second Chance

"I thought if I got Larry a job our relationship would be better," Becca wrote in a letter dated October 9, 2005. She described a time, just months after her June 1993 release from CHO, when Larry was without work, they were on public aid, and her hands shook while her brain took in medications. For help, Becca turned to Aunt Linda and Uncle Chuck, who owned a landscaping business in Baltimore, Ohio; it was a small, family-owned business started decades earlier by Chuck's father. "They hauled rock from the quarries and needed help," Becca said. "Maybe they would hire Larry. I was trying to make things better with my husband and I was getting away from my mother. Two for one. I guess that's what I thought."

All eight of them – Larry, Becca, her parents, and four children – filled a 1989 maroon Dodge minivan and drove eastward on Interstate 74 to Interstate 70 until they reached Baltimore, a small town thirty miles southeast of Columbus. Larry began working at Aunt Linda and Uncle Chuck's landscaping business while Becca and her family returned to Illinois. Weeks later, in October 1993, Larry rented one of two apartments in Baltimore, in an older white-frame house with a large front porch where kids could play or parents could sit and watch the occasional car drive past on a busy day. Becca and her two-year-old daughter, Alyssa, who had Larry's eyes and Becca's smile, were joined there by three-year-old Chris, whose thick dark-brown hair and deep set eyes made him the spitting image of Larry. Nathan, a blond, blue eyed four-year-old, made the trip as well, while Amanda, who was eight and looked like Becca in her childhood days, stayed in Illinois with Becca's parents.

Becca hoped for a second chance: maybe her marriage would improve, maybe they could support themselves, and maybe, just maybe, her mind would find a more gentle path. After Halloween, when they took the children trick-or-treating, Becca's and Aunt Linda's families drew names for Christmas, and Becca cleaned her aunt's house for gift money. They were a family.

But things quickly changed. During the winter months, when the landscaping business was closed, Larry stayed home and drew unemployment checks; Becca spent time with her aunt sewing curtains and a bedspread for her children's room. Becca remembered how Larry was threatened by her relationship with

Cherry Blossoms & Barren Plains

Aunt Linda. "Larry said that I loved my family more than him." The fights between Becca and Larry increased, the house was a mess, and although Becca took her medications, she sensed that something was wrong. "I felt myself going manic," she later said. "Larry and I got into another fight and I went after him." He left the house and went to Aunt Linda's, who called Becca and told her to meet them at the church; Aunt Linda was a religious woman who believed that God could heal Becca's ways. After pulling into a black-topped parking lot, Becca and her three children stepped from her car and entered a conference room adjacent to the church. Inside the room was a large rectangular-shaped table with Larry, Aunt Linda, Uncle Chuck, and Brenda, a young attorney who had befriended Becca and claimed to be a Christian, standing on the other side. There was a calm moment while each waited for the other to speak. Becca couldn't remember what Larry said that day; she remembers only that his words drove her to lunge across the table and grab hold of his neck. Screaming followed. Uncle Chuck hurried to break Becca's hold. Then the room became quiet as they agreed to take Becca home where she could think through her thoughts.

Becca settled the children in for the night and drew herself a hot bath. She sat in the tub that night, her thoughts began to surface: If only I could die, maybe peace would come. Minutes later, she rose from the tub and wiped off the beads of water that clung to her skin. She grabbed the blue cotton robe that hung on the bathroom door and walked across the room. There, sitting on the dresser top, was a bottle of Risperdal, an antipsychotic medication designed to quiet the mind. Becca held the bottle in her left hand, pushed down with her right, and loosened the safe-lock top. She, then, dumped a hand full of pills – some thirty in all – into her mouth and flushed them down with slow, continuous gulps of water, and lay across the bed. The voices must stop, she thought. I'm tired and Larry doesn't love me. I'd be better off dead.

Larry walked into the room and saw Becca lying on the bed. An empty bottle of Risperdal was on the bedroom floor. What have you done to yourself? he yelled, as he watched her drift to a dangerous place. He rushed to the phone, called Linda, and returned to the bed, where he held Becca in his arms and told her not to die in front of the kids.

The sound of tires rolling over their gravel driveway and the slamming of car doors broke the silent night. The front door opened, and Linda and Chuck rushed into the house. While Linda called for an ambulance, Chuck told Larry that if Becca died, it would be on him. Becca remembers fragments of what happened that night: the racing ambulance; the paramedics trying to keep her awake; and fighting the doctor as he pumped her stomach dry. Three days later, in February 1994, she awoke in a hospital bed in Lancaster, Ohio, where Uncle Chuck – a church deacon – stood over her, recited scriptures, and promised that God would show her the way.

Since the small-town hospital was ill-equipped for mental health patients, Becca was transferred to the Ohio State University hospital, located in Athens. Becca took her medications, began group therapy, and walked the hospital floor. While Linda and Chuck came to visit, Larry and the children stayed away. The sadness was strong, and the depression was persistent. Three weeks passed before Becca was released from the state hospital. Their intentions were good, but the policy was clear: medicate the patients and prepare them for the outside world as expediently as possible. Long-term therapy gave way to pharmaceutical care. But sometimes a small paper cup filled with jellybean-colored pills just won't do the job.

Becca and Larry went back to their apartment while the children stayed with Linda and Chuck; maybe Becca and Larry could mend their broken relationship. Becca's mind was consumed by the rhythm of her metronomic thoughts: I am a terrible mother. I abandoned my kids. Larry doesn't love me.

Days later, Becca was back in the state hospital. The children lived with her aunt and uncle, while Larry drove himself back to Illinois. Becca's aunt and her attorney-friend Brenda suggested that she sign a thirty-five dollar form that transferred the guardianship of her three children to Aunt Linda and Uncle Chuck. Now that her husband was gone and she had given her children away, Becca fell into a bad depression, a can't-move depression.

Three weeks passed before Becca was released. She moved in with her aunt and uncle and was told to find a job and get her life in order. "I was so tired," Becca later said. "The medicine was kicking my butt." She was not allowed to be alone with her children and was monitored by her aunt, who pushed pills of every color. Often times, Becca disappeared for the day; she remembers going to the local movie house and watching *The Three Musketeers* three times in a row. "I just stared at the movie screen. I felt myself going nuts."

The next day, Becca was talking on the telephone with Brenda and spoke of troubled times: the sadness of Larry moving away; the absence of private time with her children; and an off-the-cuff remark about how she might be better off if she left her children and moved back to Illinois. Upon hearing the conversation, Aunt Linda grabbed at the phone, trying to pull it away. A scuffle followed as Becca hit her aunt in the head with the receiver. Becca thought that it was not a serious blow. Still, it was enough for Linda to call the police, who came to the house and found Becca sitting on a dark bedroom floor, singing and rocking back and forth as she held her three children. The police broke her grip on the children, secured her wrists with metal handcuffs, and took her to the Lancaster hospital, where she was sedated and transferred to the state hospital instead of jail.

"This was worse than before," Becca later said. "They threw me in with the psychos. The murderers, the schizos, the whole kit-and-kaboodle." Becca was isolated and denied any contact with her family. She remembers only her meaningless walks up and down the hospital halls. "I did thirty days there and was scared straight for sure." Upon her release, she was moved from the state hospital to the jail, where she waited four hours before a hearing with the judge. Aunt Linda, who had a restraining order against Becca, and Brenda were at the hearing, hoping to prolong Becca's jail time and to keep the children. But early into the hearing, it became obvious that Brenda was not licensed to practice law in Ohio. "Brenda lied," Becca said. "The judge held Brenda in contempt and told her to shut up and sit down. The guardianship papers were invalid and I was released for time served."

Because of a restraining order and six months probation, Becca could not go to her aunt's and see her children. She was left on the courthouse steps where she waited for her brother to take her to his home. It was there that she did what she dreaded most – called her mother and asked for help. Like many times before, her parents imagined that Becca, somehow, had messed things up again. "My parents paid the court costs so I could leave Ohio and the balance on the Fashion Bug Credit Card so Larry's mother would not press charges." In April 1994, Becca and the children moved back to Illinois and lived with her parents; Larry stayed with his parents as well.

***

On April 10, 2006, Becca wrote about a sleepless night when memories broke fast. It was about an earlier time in 1992 when troubled thoughts were tamped down until they became hard and repressed for nearly fourteen years. Just months before her first admission to CHO, she had run away from Larry and the children. "The doctors thought I did it because of the stress and all of my fighting with Larry. But there's more to it," Becca said. At the time, Becca worked two jobs, cleaned the house, cooked the meals, and cared for the children. Larry worked one job but would not care for the children when he was home. "He wouldn't do anything," Becca claimed. "I had to get a baby sitter to watch the kids when I left for my second job." On one such night when Becca came home, she asked Larry to help give the children a bath. When he refused, Becca climbed into the bathtub with the four children. "I was exhausted and couldn't stop crying," she said. "I remember staring at the kids and thinking that I should drown them all and kill myself." Becca said she didn't know what stopped her that night, but a week later she went to work and didn't come back. "Maybe I knew subconsciously that I needed to get away or something very bad was coming down. I guess I'm lucky that what happened in 1998 didn't happen in 1992."

This chilling revelation had never touched the ears of another person. As I read her words, I felt the hopelessness that squashed and squeezed her will to live. If only things could have been different, I thought. If she could have lived during a time of compassion for the mentally ill when long-term care was the order of the day. There was, perhaps, a better time: the late eighteenth and early nineteenth centuries, before support for the mental health community had mutated into an environment where more people like Becca are incarcerated in prisons rather than housed in hospitals for the mentally ill. Now, in 2006, the National Alliance for the Mentally Ill (NAMI) reports that 16 percent of the prison population is severely mentally ill and fits the psychiatric classification for illnesses such as schizophrenia, major depression, and bipolar disorder. Twenty-five percent of the local jail populations are mentally ill, and when you factor in other mental illness and substance abuse, the numbers exceed fifty percent.

But what was considered state-of-the-art treatment for the mentally ill changed over time. According to Joseph J. Mehr in *An Illustrated History of Illinois Public Mental Health Services: 1847 to 2000*, the nation's population of patients in state hospitals and asylums grew from 8,500 to 18,000 in the decade following 1870. The numbers continued to double each decade until 1900, when the nation treated nearly 150,000 patients. Natural population growth, immigration, and the belief that long-term therapy could cure the mentally ill, all contributed to an expansion that would, in time, change the national outlook from the optimistic to the overwhelmed.

By the late 1920's, the number of mental hospitals in Becca's home state, Illinois, had grown to nine: Jacksonville, Elgin, Anna, Kankakee, Chester, East Moline, Peoria, Chicago, and Alton. In 1927, construction began on the Manteno State Hospital, the tenth such hospital in Illinois. The patients in Illinois hospitals and asylums had grown from 22,282 in 1930 to 35,852 in 1950; the depression and a world war reduced legislative support; the over-crowded and under-staffed hospitals became scandalous, not only in Becca's home state, but throughout the nation; and the 1960's produced seven times more patients than staff. It became apparent that curing the mentally ill sometimes required long periods of treatment and, in some cases, was unattainable. The mental health community tested new techniques as they sought a short-cut or an instant cure for their patients: fever and insulin shock treatments; convulsive, occupational and industrial therapies; eltro shock, hydrotherapy, water packs and sprays. Nearly 1,000 lobotomies were performed in Illinois, alone.

Unlike other drugs that relied on heavy sedation, chlorpromazine (Thorazine) – one of the most commonly prescribed psychotropic drugs of the 1960's – was effective in reducing the symptoms of psychosis. In a brief period of one or two years, the drug found favor with American psychiatrists, and other medications were developed for specific illnesses such as depression, mania, and anxiety. The antipsychotic medications calmed the patient, making him or her more receptive to psychotherapy. Pharmaceutical progress and the social stigma of mental hospitals perpetuated through books like *The Snake Pit,* by Mary Jane Ward, and movies like *One Flew Over the Cuckcoo's Nest*, adapted from the book by Ken Kesey, encouraged depopulation in the mental hospitals. Deinstitutionalization and community-based programs were the key words of the day.

***

That octopus-like creature – the one that I imagined – had

sprayed Becca's mind with homicidal thoughts. On August 3, 1994, Becca checked into the emergency room at the Community Hospital of Ottawa and claimed that she was overwhelmed with a desire to kill her mother. Like many times before, Becca had been fighting with her mother, her husband, and feeling the stress of raising four children. Two months earlier, she had stopped taking her medications, saying that she could better deal with the stress when off medications. Now, her mania had switched to a deep depression and her anger was just beneath her skin.

Archibald Hutchinson, M.D., the admitting physician, recorded her psychiatric history. In summary, Hutchinson states that the patient believes that her biological mother was very detached, and physically, as well as verbally, abusive. The patient was mostly raised by grandparents, and stated that she helped raise her younger brother. Patient admits to a longstanding history of multiple bouts of depression, swinging from baseline mood to severe depression, as well as uncontrollable anger outbursts where the patient states she "loses it." These episodes are marked by depression or irritability, and gets her into multiple fights. Patient states that parents had recently left for West Virginia to take care of maternal grandmother who was very sick, and while gone, the patient had taken care of the house cleaning, mowing the grass, and at that time Larry, the patient's second husband, was with her. Upon return, mother accused Becca of stealing $400.00 in quarters. Patient finally had an irresistible anger outburst, and felt that she was going to kill her parents, which caused present hospitalization. Patient has been on multiple medications in the past, including Lithium Carbonate, Buspar, Wellbutrin, Prozac, Pamelor, Tegretol, Corgard, Tranxene, Haldol and Artane. Patient describes her husband, Larry, as unemployed, an alcoholic and a drug addict since he was 12-years-of age, verbally abusive, very selfish, narcissistic personality.

Patient did well during her hospitalization and the staff noted her contributions to the group. On August 31 it was felt that the patient was sufficiently stabilized and was not homicidal or a danger to herself and in need of further inpatient hospitalization. Patient is discharged to self. Medication on discharge: Tegretol 300 mg 3x per day, Prozac 20 mg in the morning. Patient is to follow-up with her long-time therapist and to attend an out-patient program on Tuesdays evenings from 7:00 to 8:00 p.m. Prognosis is fair secondary to good improvement during this hospitalization.

Cherry Blossoms & Barren Plains

In a little white house down by the river.

"His name was James." That's what Becca called him as we sat in the visit room at the Dwight Correctional Center. "I don't know if it was rape, abuse, or if we were just in love." Becca's medical records showed that when she was a young girl, she was raped by a family member, and was later diagnosed with Post Traumatic Stress Disorder. Now, some 26 years after that haunting summer, Becca searched for a label. "I've never thought of it as rape," she said. "I was willing and it was something I enjoyed." But after she told me her story, she was not so sure.

It was the summer of 1980. Becca was 14 and James was 19. "He was my first cousin and always looked after me. When I was eight, he even showed me how to put a worm on a fishing hook." Six summers later, while Becca's brother passed the summer in West Virginia and her parents worked, she and James spent secluded days in Becca's home – a small, three-bedroom frame house with burnt-red siding, located in Streator, Illinois in a quiet, mind-your-own-business neighborhood. Several months earlier, James had suffered a hunting accident, when a defective safety allowed his gun to misfire and blow a third of his foot away. Now, this tall, two-hundred-pound slab of a man hobbled on one leg. He just wanted to heal and collect a generous settlement from the gun manufacturer.

Each day, Becca applied an ointment and changed the bandage on his tender foot, prepared his meals, and drew his bath. "It was like we were married. I cared for him and he was nice to me." The two of them rested on the living room floor and watched their favorite television programs. On one such day, Becca recalled, James slid next to her and gave her an unfamiliar kiss. She was accustomed to the hugs and the wrestling on the floor, but this was different. She jumped from the floor and raced to her bedroom and locked the door, where she stayed for the rest of the day.

James later apologized and said that it was okay for him to kiss her; after all, he cared about her and wanted to share his affection. But we might never know if he loved her or if he was a hunter stalking his prey, for days later, the kisses returned, kisses that were longer, deeper, and wetter than before. "It was something I began to like," she said. The kissing moved to the touching and stroking of places on her body where she had never experienced touch before, and finally, to the most intimate act: they made love nearly every day. Becca continued to make his meals and care for his wound, and James continued to show her a new reality. He would find a state where they could get married, draw from the lucrative settlement that was certain to come, and live in a little white house down by the river.

At the end of the summer, Becca went back to high school, her brother returned to their quiet home in Streator, and James joined his family in North Dakota. The two of them, Becca and James, communicated through letters and telephone calls that left her parents with troubling bills. Besides the emotional devastation his absence brought, Becca felt quite ill – fatigue and nausea filled her days. She was hospitalized and the doctors searched for the cause of her illness. Urine and blood tests were followed by an ultrasound which showed the beginnings of an unborn child. Becca was pregnant.

While she searched her confused mind, her fears were allayed by his vow: James loves me and we're going to get married and live on his big settlement and having a baby will be great. But Becca's parents did not share her enthusiasm. They listened with closed ears and stared with rigid eyes while Becca told them about her wonderful summer, when she and James fell in love. They turned and walked out of the hospital room and never spoke of that summer again. They pushed the knowledge deep into some distant crevice of their cerebral cortices, where unwanted memories are thrown away.

A nurse who lived in their neighborhood made arrangements for Becca to have an abortion. "My parents told me that I was going to have some medical tests," Becca said. Days later, while she sat in a doctor's office someplace in Wisconsin, a fair-skinned motherly-looking nurse entered the room and told her about the abortion and how it would be done. *Why should I have an abortion?* Becca thought. *This is our baby. We're going to get married and live off the big settlement. Everything will be just as we planned.* Becca's face tightened as she refused to sign the consent form. She insisted on calling James, who said that the decision was up to her. "He never said if I should or should not have the abortion." Since James was her first cousin, the medical staff convinced Becca that there might be some problems with the baby. "That's when I decided to have the abortion," she said.

What else happened in the office that day is somewhat of a blur. Becca doesn't remember where the office was located, only that she thought it was in Wisconsin, and she doesn't remember how they aborted her baby. I can only imagine that like most abortions, they gave her a local or general anesthetic. They probably dilated her cervix so the contents of her uterus could pass out of her body. They might have used a hand-held syringe or a small-bore tube attached to a suction machine – back in 1980 it was more than likely a syringe – and pulled the chunk of flesh from her insides. There was probably some blood, but in a few minutes, it was over. Yet when she left the office that day, her world would never be the same as what James promised her when they lay together on the living room floor.

It was some three years later, when Becca was 17 and James was 22, that the two of them first saw each other at a family reunion. Although she resisted going, her parents insisted that she attend, and like they had done for the past three years, they pretended that what was sucked from her uterus that summer was not a baby at all. "I always felt like I received all of the blame," Becca said. "It was all my fault." Just as before, no one, including James, ever talked about that summer, and how his promise was never kept – that they would get married, live off the big settlement, and have their baby. Even into the early part of Becca's prison term, she received a few letters from James and, like before, he never mentioned his promise.

Now, as we sat in the visit room, I continued to marvel at how Becca's parents and James had forgotten the unforgettable summer. "I find it difficult to imagine that no one ever talked about what happened that summer?" I asked.

"No one ever said a word," she answered.

"Not even James?" I asked.

"Not even James," she answered.

"Do you know that in Illinois what James did is considered a crime?" I asked. I had checked the Illinois Criminal Code and discovered that a sexual act is considered a criminal assault if the person has sexual penetration with another person who is less than 18 years of age and is a family member, or sexual penetration with a non-family member who is at least 13 but under 18, and the defendant is over the age of 17 and in a position of trust. It is considered a class I felony with a mean sentence of 5 years in prison.

Becca seemed a bit surprised by my remark. "Well, it's still hard for me to know what to call it," she said. "I don't know if it was rape or not."

"What would you have done if that girl had been your daughter who was 14 and had sex with her first cousin who was 19, and then became pregnant and had an abortion?" I asked.

Her face stiffened as she answered, "I'd kick his ass."

Cherry Blossoms & Barren Plains

"I just needed more help."

Many years later, on August 31, 1994, and after Becca's release from CHO, she moved into a motel that hugged a busy street in downtown Streator. It was your typical motel room – two small chairs, a double bed, a television, a desk, a bathroom, and tucked away in the top drawer of the night stand, a Gideon Bible that promised a better life. Since Becca was not a threat to herself or to another person, she was released with instructions to continue taking her medications, report back to the hospital's psychiatrist every two weeks, and have limited contact with her family. The medical staff at CHO acknowledged the improvement that Becca had made while in a more controlled environment and suggested that she spend the next few weeks in a local motel. The children would stay with Larry at his parents' home.

Becca would have preferred staying in CHO or another mental hospital for a longer period of time – maybe two years, Becca later said – where she would have worked on her problems and lived in a more tranquil world. "I just needed more help," she said. But long-term care in a state hospital was a thing of the past. The mental health community had moved from the long-term care of the early twentieth century, to the overcrowded state hospitals in the 1950s that were filled to over 150% of capacity, to the community-based mental health facilities that began in the 1960s. The census of state hospitals in Illinois had dropped from 36,000 patients in 1960 to 18,000 in 1970, and the 1980s saw budget cuts responsible for closing hospitals and cutting administrative staff in community centers. In the 1990s, patients in the Illinois mental health facilities and state hospitals declined from 3500 in 1990, to 1800 by the end of the decade. In 1994, the ninety-minute program or the Zone Center program, as it was called, sought to provide a local, multi-service mental health facility within a 90 minute drive for each person seeking short-term, out-patient care.

The transition from State Mental Hospitals to the Community Health Centers reached maturation by the enactment of the Community Mental Health Center Act, (CMHC), in 1963, when many psychiatrists believed that long-term treatment promoted, rather than reduced, chronic mental illness. Improved therapy and psychotic drugs, they believed, could eliminate the need for long-term care, and thus, the need for state mental hospitals. Legislators, longing for a more cost-effective approach, jumped on the community approach as well.

In 1955, Congress had asked the National Institute for Mental Health, (NIMH), to appoint a joint commission to examine the treatment of mental illness. Rather that abandon state mental hospitals, the commission endorsed moral therapy, a philosophical idea of an earlier age. They wanted a system of small treatment-intensive hospitals, limited to 200 beds each, one community mental health center (CMHC) for each 50,000 residents, double federal spending in five years, and triple in ten years. It was not the recommendation that the psychiatric and legislative communities sought.

With the election of President John F. Kennedy, a long-time advocate for the mentally ill, the earlier joint commission report was revived. Kennedy appointed a Secretary's committee consisting of the Secretary of Health, Education and Welfare, the Secretary of Labor, and others from the NIMH to study the joint commission's recommendations. There was a shared consensus that the strengthening of the communities, social welfare, and educational programs would correct the harsh environment that Kennedy later declared to be responsible for mental retardation and mental illness. The newly formed committee emphasized prevention and a substantial reduction in the number of state mental hospitals. Gone was moral therapy and the NIMH's earlier recommendation for a system of small treatment-intensive state hospitals.

The Secretary's report to President Kennedy recommended the implementation of one community mental health clinic for each 50,000 residents, with eight essential services, including rehabilitation programs and supervision of foster home care for discharged patients. In his message to congress, Kennedy, too, included rehabilitation and foster home care as key elements of a comprehensive community mental health center. But when the NIMH drew up the final regulations, they dropped the earlier recommendation of the joint commission that "after-care and rehabilitation are essential parts of all service to mental patients, and the various methods of achieving rehabilitation should be integrated in all forms of service." NIMH listed five requirements that each center had to meet in order to qualify for federal funds: inpatient services, partial hospitalization, outpatient services, twenty-four hour emergency, and consultation and educational programs.

Rael Jean Isaac & Virginia C. Armat in <u>Madness in the Streets:</u>

Cherry Blossoms & Barren Plains

<u>How Psychiatry and the Law Abandoned the Mentally Ill</u>, lay much of the responsibility for society's neglect of the chronic mentally ill upon the psychiatrists of the mid 1960's, who viewed long-term stays in mental hospitals as the problem rather than the solution. Their efforts, in part, left the schizophrenics and those like Becca who suffered with bipolar disorder, to roam the streets, fill the jails, and sometimes live with families unable to deal with the demands of mental illness.

***

    Becca was not alone at the motel on that summer day in 1994. When Becca moved in, James, an older, heavy-set friend with thinning hair, whom she had met at CHO, stayed with her for one week until he found a way to his home in Columbus, Ohio. John and Deanna, two more friends from CHO, came to Becca's motel room almost every day; Deanna brought her three children as well. John was a small, quiet, skinny guy with a heck of a temper, while blond, blue-eyed Deanna was out-going. Larry and their four children made daily visits. While Deanna drank, looked for available men, and urged Becca to take that path, Larry told Becca that she had to choose between him and her newly-found friends. Becca chose her friends.
    New men filtered into her life. One night when Larry dropped by a local bar, like he had done many times before, he found Becca with a man named Dave. The men fought long and hard that night until their bodies were covered in sweat, and blood ran from their noses. The next day Becca and her children moved into her parents' home, while they were in West Virginia taking care of her grandmother. No more than two sunsets passed before her friends from CHO – John and Deanna, the one with three children – moved in with Becca. By this time, Larry was not speaking to Becca, and his parents told him that if he moved in with Becca, they would not speak to him again.
    The swings between mania and depression are common symptoms of bipolar disorder, and for Becca the movements were swift. This, added to a stress-filled environment, pushed Becca into her can't-move depression. Days went by when she wanted to die. She told her friends to move out of the house and begged Larry to come back and live with her. Life without Larry, the only man she truly loved, was not worth living. After she promised to take her

medications and to keep her doctor appointments, Larry agreed to find an apartment where the two of them and the four children could live like a real family.

But the happiness was brief and the pattern was clear. It was a movie seen many times before: Larry did not work, Becca and the children were on public aid, and Larry accused her of spending too much time with her friends. The fighting increased. At times, the children hovered in a corner of the room and choked off their sadness. They became the "quiet" children. "You could see the fear in their eyes," Becca later said. One such incident was the time when Becca and Larry were fighting and Becca fell down the stairs. "I honestly don't know if he pushed me or if I just fell," Becca said. "All I know is that I couldn't walk for a few days and ended up having surgery. Larry wouldn't take care of me. I had to hire someone." Weeks later, when Becca was on her feet and Christmas was near, a friend told Becca that she saw Larry with another woman at the local bar. "We took the kids and went to the bar. Sure enough, Larry was with another woman. I didn't say anything. We just left." Later that night, while Becca and her children sat in the apartment and listened to Christmas carols, Larry rushed through the open door. He screamed, cocked-back his fist, and threatened to bust her in the face. The "quiet" children listened and watched their Christmas tree fall to the wooden floor. "I remember the hate in his eyes that night. I knew it was over for the two of us."

During the first half of 1995, their relationship was dominated by fighting and a feeling of hopelessness. Becca lied to Larry, telling him that she was going out with a friend, when, in reality, she went to a local bar and drank alone. "My parents moved to West Virginia for good," Becca said. "Then I had no one." In early May, Becca kicked Larry out of their apartment and later met Ciro, a shy, dark-skinned Mexican with a fierce temper, who hung out at the local bar. "We began sleeping together," Becca later said. "Larry had a girlfriend too." While Ciro worked for the railroad and came home only on weekends, Becca spent the days at the local bar and the nights with different men.

"When you slept with so many men," I asked, "did you think it was wrong?" Becca hesitated before answering, as if it was the first time she had thought about its rightness or wrongness. "I don't think I ever thought about it. I was so manic that I just didn't care."

Becca was writing bad checks to support her drinking habit and had stopped taking her medications. When she asked Larry to take care of the kids, his girlfriend told him to stay away. When Larry agreed to pick up the kids, they waited for hours on the front porch. "There were times when me and the kids went downtown and saw Larry with his girlfriend. We'd chase him in our car, but he always got away."

Becca had filed for divorce but Larry wouldn't sign the papers. A friend, who owned a local bar, hired Becca as a part-time bartender and introduced her to Mario, a tall, well-built man whom Becca described as "mighty fine," followed by a shy chuckle. Jaun and Shane, two boys in their late teens, stayed with her children while she went out with Mario. "All I had to do was buy them a case of beer. The kids really liked them."

When Becca was arrested for writing bad checks and placed in jail, Larry went to the apartment and took the children to his parents' house. Hours later, Amanda's Grandma and Grandpa, the parents of Becca's first husband, bailed her out. But when Becca left the jail, she never picked up the children. "I needed a break from them and I felt sick. I had been off my meds and had been leaving the kids with whoever would take them." Now, Becca was hanging out at a Mexican bar and sleeping with anyone who showed an interest. She had seemingly lost her soul. Peter D. Kramer describes such behavior as "rapid cycling." Kramer, author of "*Listening to Prozac: A Psychiatrist Explores Antidepressant Drugs and the Remaking of the Self,*" considers "rapid cycling" as the "gravest mood disorder." "These people may shift back and forth from deep depression to startling euphoria or to extreme irritability, sometimes in a matter of days or even hours." Kramer explains that the initial mood swings are probably triggered by trauma, but as time passes, the slightest irritant brings on an episode. And sometimes, it happens without any provocation at all. These patients can be difficult to treat, and tend to end up in a mental institution. When later asked about her behavior, Becca shook her head and said, "I couldn't think straight. I was just trying to survive."

When Larry tried to return the children, Becca stayed away. She later said that Larry went to the police and told them that he didn't want the children. "That's when I went to pick them up," Becca said. "I didn't want DCFS to take my kids." Larry and his girlfriend left for Colorado to "get away from me and start a new life. That's what Larry's parents said." Step by step, her life was falling apart. She was off her medication, out of money, her parents were living in West Virginia, and she faced possible prison time for writing bad checks. Mario found out about Ciro and the other men Becca was sleeping with, and quickly broke her nose. Shane and Juan were still coming by when Ciro was gone. "When I got home at night, me and the boys drank beer, smoked pot, and had sex."

As crazy as she was, Becca knew that she needed to find a safe place for her children. She told Amanda to stay with her biological father, and asked her mother to take her other children.

> *Two days later, she sent my uncle to pick up the kids. While the kids were in school, I disappeared and went to Decatur. I ran because I couldn't face my kids. I had let them down and abandoned them. I called and asked Amanda's grandma to keep the kids for the night. My uncle was in Streator by 10:00 a.m. the next day. This was November 17, 1995. I had to go to the lawyer's office to sign over the guardianship of my kids to my uncle and his wife. I went back to the house and packed the kids' clothes and toys and loaded the van. All I could do was cry and hug them. I had to take them to Larry's mom and dad to say goodbye. That was the worst day of my life. They were little and all they thought about was living with grandma and grandpa, and all I could think about was killing myself. As they pulled off, I threw up, and on my inside, I was dead. It was time for God to punish me for what I had done to them. My uncle told my mom that watching me give up my kids, was the worst thing he ever had to witness and he would never do it again.*
>
> *A letter from Becca dated May 14, 2006.*

Becca moved out of her apartment and began living with Ciro. Although her body was marked with black eyes and multiple bruises, she stayed with him. "Each time he threatened to leave me, I begged him to stay. I was more afraid of being alone than the beatings. On December 15, 1995, my divorce was final. Since Ciro wanted to be an American citizen, he married me on December 19, 1995. On our wedding night, he beat the crap out of me."

Ciro left the railroad and found a job washing dishes at a restaurant in Olgesby, a thirty mile drive from Streator. While Ciro was gone, Becca invited the boys – Juan and Shane – to come over and party. On one night, when Ciro came home earlier than before, he kicked everyone out of the apartment. "He beat me unconscious that night and Amanda saw it all."

Becca described a night in February of 1996, when Becca, Ciro, Ciro's uncle, and Pam, the next door neighbor, were sitting around the kitchen table and drinking some beer. "All of a sudden he threw a glass at me and broke my front tooth and busted my chin open. When I asked him why he hit me, he started punching me in the face." Later that night, Becca claims that Ciro wanted to have sex. When she refused, he hit her, raped her, and finally, he passed out. The next day, Becca called work and said that she was sick. When her boss came by to check on her, she begged Becca to leave Ciro. "I couldn't leave," Becca said. "I believed that God was punishing me for all of the bad things that I had done."

It was September 1996 when she first met Chad, the man who would later become her fourth husband. At first, it was just a one-night stand, like she had with other men before. One month later, around 2:00 a.m., Chad showed up at her front door, trying to convince Becca to leave with him. Chad's pleas woke Ciro, who was drunk and had been passed out on the bathroom floor. When he stormed towards the open door, Chad drove away. "I remember Ciro hitting me as hard as he could that night," Becca said.

Chad began coming by the apartment when Ciro was at work. "He told me that he was married and that he was unhappy." One morning in November, when Ciro came back to the house for something that he had forgotten, he found Chad and Becca in bed. In a fit of rage, Ciro ran to the kitchen and grabbed a black-handled knife from the cabinet drawer. He gripped the handle hard and pushed the blade into Chad's arm, and with a second thrusting blow, he pushed it deep into Chad's stomach. He turned and swung the knife wildly as he moved toward Becca. As she raised her hands to protect her face, the knife penetrated the back of her hands. "My hands felt like they were on fire," she later said. Chad crawled to his truck and drove to the hospital, where he told the police what had happened. When the police arrived at Becca's apartment, Ciro had sped away. They took Becca to the local hospital where the two of them, Chad and Becca, were treated for their wounds. Days later, Ciro went to the police and turned himself in. A plea agreement was reached that required Ciro to spend the next four months in jail.

***

Images of Becca's path from 1994 to 1998, which led to the murder of her five-year-old step-daughter, stick to my mind like old wallpaper. Becca was hospitalized on five different occasions; four were voluntary and one was involuntary, when she hit her aunt in the head with a telephone receiver. While the doctors recognized Becca's improvement in the controlled environment of a state mental hospital, her longest stay was barely one month. She was diagnosed with bipolar illness and borderline personality disorder, and, at times, had homicidal thoughts. But each time, she was released back into her abusive world. Long term care in a state mental hospital would have provided proper monitoring of her medications and the development of the coping skills needed to deal with her mental illness.

History shows the logic that led to the deinstitutionalization of our mental health system, and hindsight allows us to decide whether our society moved too far and too fast in one direction. In the 1960s, when the population of state mental hospitals was bursting at the seams, and when our national budget was stretched by a rapid population growth and the psychological damage from the Vietnam war, an estimated thirty-five thousand troops were psychiatric casualties, America longed for a quick solution that would cure the mentally ill and empty the hospital beds. The success of the pharmaceutical drugs of the 1960s, the ensuing budget cuts, and claims that hospitals had become warehouses for the mentally ill, led to the depopulation of our mental hospitals and a move towards community-controlled mental health centers. While supporters of the movement were many, opponents saw it as the premature and dangerous dismantling of our mental health system.

If we follow the money, we can see the current that carried the financial burden from the federal government to the states, and back again to the federal government. In 1965, with the enactment of Medicaid and Medicare, a cloud hung over mental health care. Medicaid specifically excluded payments for patients in state psychiatric hospitals and other "institutions for mental diseases" – a hospital, nursing facility, or other institution of more than 16 beds, that is primarily engaged in providing diagnosis, treatment, or care of persons with mental diseases, including medical attention, nursing care, and related services, 42 U.S.C. &1396d(i). While Medicaid treated a host of illnesses for people between the ages of 21 to 65, some 470,000 individuals receiving inpatient psychiatric care were forgotten. The objective was clear: to accelerate deinstitutionalization, and to shift the costs back to the states.

Most of the mentally ill patients, like Becca, were indigent and lacked private insurance to pay for their care; states were left to pick up the bills. But states found a way to transfer the costs back to the federal government. If the psychiatric patients were moved from state mental hospitals to nursing homes, general hospitals, or other facilities covered by Medicaid, the state eliminated their costs, and received Medicaid payments of somewhere between 50 and 80 percent of the costs incurred at the Medicaid approved facilities. The fact that mental health care treatment was inferior, or lacked any rehabilitation program, was of little concern.

We have moved large numbers of the mentally ill from state mental hospitals to the streets of major cities, where they eat from garbage cans and we look the other way. Rich Lowry, editor of *National Review*, wrote in a July 31, 2003 editorial that "there are some 450,000 homeless people in the United States, and about a third are mentally ill... Most of the mentally ill roaming the streets are too sick to know they are sick. Roughly 50 percent of schizophrenics and those with bipolar disorder do not know they are mentally ill." Prisons are filled with the once-feared, now forgotten mentally ill. According to Fuller Torrey, president of the Treatment Advocacy Center, "The Los Angeles County jail, with 3,400 mentally ill prisoners, is de facto the largest psychiatric inpatient facility in the United States. New York's Rikers Island jail, with 2,800 mentally ill prisoners, is the second-largest."

Lowry reports that in 1955 there were 559,000 people in state psychiatric hospitals. Today there are fewer than 50,000. If the numbers had grown in proportion to the national population growth, we would have more than 900,000 people in today's state hospitals. The decreased numbers are maintained, in large part, by the legal difficulty of having someone involuntarily committed into a mental hospital. The battle persists between those who carry the banner for the civil liberties of the mentally ill, and those who advocate the involuntary commitment of someone who suffers from a major mental illness.

Pete Earley, author of *Crazy: A Father's Search Through America's Mental Health Madness,* gives a gripping account of mental health care in the United States. As a journalist and father of a son who has bipolar illness, he offers a fresh perspective on why it is so difficult for someone to receive long-term care in a mental hospital. Earley felt the anger that other parents experience when their child was refused mental heath treatment at a hospital emergency room. When his son was clearly delusional and refused to recognize his illness, Earley was unable to have him involuntarily committed. To do so would have violated his son's civil liberties, the doctors said. Patients can be involuntarily committed only if they threaten to do harm to themselves or to another person.

Earley talked with Morton Birnbaum, a general practitioner/psychiatrist and advocate for the mentally ill, who is credited as a leader of the civil rights movement that made it more difficult for a mentally ill person to be involuntarily committed to a mental hospital. When Earley asked about his motives, he was surprised by Birhbaum's response. Birhbaum never intended for his civil rights campaign to cause the results it had. His premise was straightforward; mental health patients in state hospitals have a constitutional "right to treatment," and hospitals had to treat the patients or set them free.

In the early 1960's, patients were sometimes housed in state mental hospitals for indefinite periods of time. They had been involuntarily committed by judges and relatives, and in some cases were not receiving the care that would lead to an improved mental state. Critics claimed that the hospitals had become warehouses for the mentally ill, and that the patients were quickly forgotten. Birhbaum was not trying to close the hospital doors; he was demanding proper care. Several attorneys successfully utilized Birhbaum's legal premise that patients have a "right to treatment," and demanded that hospitals spend millions of dollars on their legal obligation, or close their doors. Massive financial burdens drove many legislators to choose the latter, to close the doors, and move towards a policy of deinstitutionalization. Civil liberties for the mentally ill became the overriding issue.

In the twenty-first century, long-term care is history. Today, in 2006, a typical stay in a mental hospital lasts five days, or seven days if you're lucky. Psychopharmacology has replaced psychotherapy. Time is money. Insurance companies, health maintenance organizations, Medicare and Medicaid, continue to reduce patient reimbursements. Treatment is dictated by level of violence – is the patient a threat to himself or others – rather than the extent of one's illness. As Alex Beam, author of *Gracefully Insane: Life and Death Inside America's Premier Mental Hospital,* explains, "Today's psychiatrist must stabilize, diagnose, treat – usually with drug prescriptions – and release a disturbed man or woman in less than a week..." Follow-up visits last from 5 to15 minutes and cover such questions as, *Are you hearing any voices? Do you have dry mouth? Are you experiencing any side effects?* followed by possible alterations of the initial prescription.

There's a momentary silence, as the two of us, Becca and I, sit at our table in the visit room. Today, she has make-up on, and her lips are accented with a light shade of red that brings out the color of her hair. Her hands move in a continuous tremor. Her medication, recently changed to Lithium, causes her to shake. In 1994, when she first tried Lithium, she gained some one hundred pounds; this time, she lost twenty-one pounds. Finding the proper medication is an ongoing process. I look at her blue eyes that, at times, seem to stray into another world, and I marvel at the things Becca must see. Her stories of sadness wear me down. I ask her if anyone, during the peak of her illness tried to have her committed to a state mental hospital for long-term care, maybe for a period of one to two years.

"No," she answers. "My family and friends knew that something was wrong with me, but they didn't know what to do."

"How would you have felt if they had locked you up for a couple of years?"

"I think that I would have been fine with that," she answers. "I knew something was wrong with me and I wanted help." Still, I wondered. Today she is rational and able to exercise logic. Would she have made that decision when she was at the height of her craziness, or would she have needed someone to step forward and have her involuntarily committed into a mental hospital for long-term care? She knew "something" was wrong, but she didn't know the extent of her illness. As Lowry said, "some 50 percent of schizophrenics and those with bipolar disorder do not know they are mentally ill."

***

It was another time, the summer of 2006. Each Tuesday at 7:00 p.m., Becca and I talked for 30 minutes over the telephone. Days later, she would send a letter that addressed the topic we had discussed. I made trips to the Dwight Correctional Center where we leaned across the small round table in the visit room, and wondered what had pushed Becca down her dreadful path. "I need to understand what happened to me," Becca said. "Maybe my story can help others."

We talked about the complexities of her illness and the difficulties in making a correct diagnosis, and how her condition was more complicated than the classic Bipolar I as described in Patty Duke and Gloria Hochman's "*A Brilliant Madness: Living with Manic-Depressive Illness.*" Bipolar I, sometimes referred to as manic-depressive disorder, has the classic highs where the patient feels invincible and explodes with energy and needs only a sliver of sleep. Speech is a string of words that move fast and blur into a continuous tone. Becca remembered sitting down with a pad of paper where she recorded her thoughts, hoping to slow down her brain. In a manic state, the patient might do outrageous things, like go on an uncontrollable spending spree, make an outlandish decision, or engage in hyper-sexual activities with multiple partners. There were times when Becca went to the local bar and brought several men home to have sex throughout the night. "It was nothing to have sex with four men," she said. "It was slam bam, thank you Ma'am." Sometimes elation was replaced by feelings of irritability, outrage and an intolerance of others. In a full-blown mania, the patient quite often becomes psychotic and loses touch with reality.

The lows, the deep depressions, are darker than most people can imagine, and have little resemblance to the "blue" days that all people occasionally experience. You might escape to the seclusion of a darkened bedroom and wait for death to carry you away. Or you might feel lifeless as you struggle through your daily chores. Becca knows the sadness that depression unloads, when it became more than she could endure, when suicide seemed like her only option.

Duke and Hochman described Bipolar II, often called hypomania, as less severe than the classic Bipolar I. It is the lows without the highs. The patient might experience only brief periods of a toned-down mania. Cyclothymes are the patients with mild ups and downs that last a few days and recycle rapidly. And then there is Unipolar, which is without the highs. With this debilitating depression, 15% of patients end up committing suicide.

We talked about Becca's diagnosis: Bipolar Disorder, Mixed. Her mood swings were erratic; a hodgepodge of emotions that reached up, down, and every which way, like the jerky flight of a hummingbird. Her behavior could sometimes be confused with that of a schizophrenic. In Becca's psychotic state, her words ran fast, but if you slowed them down, unlike the words from a schizophrenic, whose message is disconnected and lacks any rational thought, her speech made sense.

Becca's secondary diagnosis of Borderline Personality Disorder, as described in the Diagnostic and Statistical Manual of Mental Disorders, (DSM-IV, published in 1994) is characterized by a pervasive instability of moods, interpersonal relationships, self-image, and behavior. While a person with Bipolar Disorder may experience similar moods for weeks at a time, a person with BPD may experience intense mood swings that last for a few hours or a day at most. They may experience fears of real or imaged abandonment, intense anger or difficulty controlling anger – displays of temper, constant anger, recurrent physical fights – unstable self-image, suicidal behavior or self mutilation, and severe dissociative symptoms.

The bursts of anger, more often found in a personality disorder, and the quickness to react in a violent way were common characteristics in Becca's world. The four husbands in her life had a knee-jerk, hit-them-in-the-face mentality. Even Carolyn, Becca's mother, was known to have fits of rage. One time, while visiting Becca at the Dwight Correctional Center, Carolyn struck Becca in the face. Carolyn, Amanda, and Becca were sitting at one of the circular tables in the visit room. When Carolyn began criticizing Amanda for having a child out of wedlock and for a general lack of responsibility, Becca stepped in and told Carolyn that she was treating Amanda the same way she had been treated. After a fist-to-the-face reaction, Carolyn was escorted out of the visit room and lost visitation privileges for six months.

The causes of BPD are mixed and can create some confusion concerning the disorder's point of origin. Many researchers believe that there is an inherited biological vulnerability or a genetic susceptibility; some believe it is a dysfunction in the Limbic area of the Brain, which controls emotion; others find the disorder to be a result of physical, mental, or sexual abuse. Many of the symptoms mirror those found in abused children who have been diagnosed with Post Traumatic Stress Disorder. There is general agreement that BPD is caused by a combination of genetic risk and environmental circumstances.

"I was impossible to live with," Becca said, while reflecting on her mental illness. "I put Larry and my family through hell. Larry did some terrible things, but sometimes he still came by the apartment after we had separated, just to see if I was okay. He loved me, but just didn't know how to help me. My mother and I had our problems but she was always there for the kids. I loved her for that. And my kids. They're the real losers." We leaned back from the small round table in the visit room, hoping to catch a moment of relief. Quiet whispers hung in the air that day.

Cherry Blossoms & Barren Plains

Greek Tragedies

Becca's life was similar to the Greek tragedies that stressed the fragility of people whose emotional pain was created by a combination of human and divine actions, and exceeded anything deserved. Evidence of Greek plays can be found as early as 550 BC, and were about tragedies confined to the lives of nobility. Maybe an error of judgment or a tragic mistake led to a horrific conclusion, or perhaps it was the product of fate. In the twentieth century, the Greek tragedy, later called the modern tragedy, was expanded to include ordinary people in domestic situations. They were tragedies about folks who made terrible mistakes or were destined to suffer.

Becca was a tragic figure who made terrible mistakes – she chose bad male partners, did not take her meds, and gave in to rage and killed the one she loved. But she was also, simultaneously, a figure for whom there was a sense of the fated, that it was beyond her control, and that something awful was going to happen to her because of her illness and the violent men in her life.

It was late 1996. The play was the same, but the cast of characters had changed. Chad Bivens, part-time derelict and alcoholic, was the lover who inflicted his abuse upon Becca, the young woman with a troubled mind and promiscuous ways. At six feet one, Chad was a well built dishwater blond with blue eyes that Becca called "awesome." Tammy Bivens, the other woman, oval-shaped and some five-feet tall, with hair that defied any particular color, was married to Chad. Tammy and Chad were the parents of Dani, the five-year-old girl who later became the object of a custody battle between her parents. Ciro Floren, while still married to Becca, was serving a four month prison sentence for thrusting a knife into Chad's belly and stabbing Becca's hand. Becca's younger children – Alyssa, Chris, and Nathan – were in West Virginia with her parents, while Amanda, her oldest child, spent most of her time with Becca, and some with Al McAllister, Becca's first husband. Chad, knifed by Ciro, had recently spent a night in jail and was fined $750 for trying to stick his knife into the belly of a friend; Tammy had been hospitalized for an overdose of Tylenol; and Becca was off her medications. "Chad liked it when I was off my meds and manic," Becca later said. "The sex was good and sometimes it lasted for hours." This play opened in a two bedroom house, with white siding and green shutters, and a small concrete porch outlined with black, iron railings. Danielle, Chad's sixteen year old cousin, had just moved in. "Danielle's mom was crazy and had kicked Danielle out of their house," Becca said.

Chad and Tammy were now divorced. Becca had tried unsuccessfully to obtain Ciro's signature on their divorce papers. Months later, Chad handed a signed copy to Becca and said that they could now be married. (Becca didn't know that Chad had forged Ciro's signature until she was later charged with bigamy, a charge that cost Becca $1,500 in attorney fees to correct.) "I should have known better than to marry Chad," Becca thought. "Even on the day of our wedding, his best friend, Kevin, asked me if I knew what I was getting into. Kevin kept telling me that I didn't have to marry Chad. But I went ahead. I didn't want to be alone." On October 18, 1997, Chad and Becca were married at the Open Bible Church in Streator, Illinois.

The tragedy continued when one inconceivable scene followed another, and then another. Each time that I asked what drove her to the finale when she ended the life of someone she loved, Becca said that she didn't know. "I can't remember any one big thing that happened. I think that it was a cumulative thing that grew until I broke." Becca paused while she found another memory. "I remember the fourth of July celebration in 1998 when I thought that this was going to be my last fourth of July. I think that I knew I was going crazy."

As we sat at a round table in the visit room, I wondered what a Positron Emission Tomography, a PET scan, of Becca's brain would have shown. The scan would have been performed in a hospital nuclear medicine department by a radiologist or nuclear medicine specialist. I imagined Becca dressed in a hospital grown, lying on a cold, hard table hooked to a scanner, a camera, and a computer. A special test medicine, called a radioactive tracer, would have been injected into the large vein in her arm. The camera recorded the tracer's signals as the tracer moved through her brain tissue. The images were then transferred to the computer screen, where different colors highlighted certain brain activity. Were some neurons more active than others? Were the levels of neurotransmitters higher or lower than those recorded in a normal person? Perhaps there were images of a brain low on serotonin that led to her deep depression, and a brain low on the neurotransmitter, GABA, that led to her manic state. Maybe I would have heard the popping and cracking sounds of neurotransmitters as they jumped from one neuron to another, and the sizzling sounds of an electrical circuit as it continually misfired. Whatever the image, I'm certain that it would have shown the brain of someone destined for tragedy.

The tragic scenes were many: like the time when Becca got a job as a part time bartender at a local bar, and Chad harassed the customers each time Becca gave them a passing glance. Chad was eventually banned from the bar. Or the time when Becca and Danielle got into a fight with Chad over Dani. Chad gave Danielle a black eye and bit Becca in the face. Or the time when Tammy called and asked if Dani could come over for Christmas. "I told Chad that I wasn't going to make Dani go if she didn't want to. Chad knocked me out and called his mother. When I woke up his mother was sitting next to me. Chad's father offered to pay my plane fare to go visit my parents and children in West Virginia. He always wanted to buy me something when Chad beat me up." Or the time when Amanda called Becca at 1:00 a.m. and told her not to come home. That Chad was in bed with another woman. And the time when Tammy called DCFS and lied about Chad having sex with Danielle, his sixteen year old cousin. "When I found out," Becca said, "I got Tammy really bad. Chad kept pulling me off her and I kept going back. The police came to the house to talk to me. I said she lied and they arrested Tammy for filing a false policy report. She went to jail. I told her if she signed Dani over to us, we would bail her out. She did and we had total custody of Dani."

I asked Becca why Dani never wanted to visit her mother. Becca's voice took on a hardened tone. "Dani told me that she was afraid of Tammy's boyfriend. His name was John. She said that he was touching her in her private places. I had Dani tell her grandmother the same story. Then we called DCFS. Tammy got mad and quit calling. She ended up marrying John."

Becca quit her bartending job and began babysitting Ben, a nine-month-old baby of Paula, a friend, a victim of domestic abuse, and an alleged drug user. "I tried the drugs one time, but didn't like them," Becca said. "They brought me down and I liked my manic state much better." Now Becca spent most of her time caring for Amanda, Ben and Dani. Maybe Becca missed her younger children who were living in West Virginia. Whatever the reason, the bond between Becca and Dani grew to the point where Becca considered the blond hair, blue-eyed five-year-old to be her own. "I loved her like my own daughter," Becca said.

In the summer of 1998, Becca, Amanda, and Dani went to West Virginia to visit her parents and her three children. While in West Virginia, Dani, Becca, her children, and their two cousins all stayed in Aunt Marlene's house. "Dani thought that she was in heaven with all the kids, and they worshiped her," Becca said. "Dani began to believe that the kids were her brothers and sisters. My mom and dad fell in love with her too." One month later, Becca's parents took them back to Illinois where they stayed for a few weeks. By this time, Becca and Chad were living in a larger four bedroom house, with plenty of room for the family. Becca was hoping that they would find jobs and be financially ready to bring her children back to Illinois by the end of the year. "Before my family went back to West Virginia, Chad was beginning to dish out some of his crap. My mom begged me to let Dani go back with them, but I refused." Becca paused. "I should of let her go. If I had only known what was going to happen."

After Becca's parents returned to West Virginia, the tragic scenes returned: like the time when Chad locked Becca in the basement until the police drove away. Or the time when Becca came home and found Chad drunk and on the dining room floor with a half-naked young girl. "I took the kids and left for the night," Becca said. "The next day, Chad accused me of going out and spending the night with another man. He broke two of my ribs, my cheek bone, and cut my head open." Or the time when Chad grabbed Becca's hair, slammed her face into the living room wall, and broke her nose. Or the times when Becca called the police and told them that Chad was drunk and had Dani in the car. "It got to the point when Chad could not even pay Dani to get in the car with him. She didn't want to leave me." Or the time when Chad was so drunk that Becca wouldn't take him with her and the children for their usual Saturday night at the bowling alley. Chad called his mother and got a ride to the bowling alley. "Chad stormed into the bowling alley and began punching me. People jumped on him and called the police. Chad spent the night in jail."

By September 1998, Becca's mind eclipsed into darkness, when the cloud of mental illness cast a shadow that blocked her ability to reason. "I was on another planet," Becca said in a letter written to me on November 7, 2006. I had asked Becca to describe her mental state leading up to Dani's death. "I was here but I wasn't. People asked me if I was okay and I'd just say yes and move on. Chad wasn't working and it was driving me nuts, wondering where the next money was going to come from. I began babysitting another child. Her name was Katie. Now I had Amanda and Dani, and I was babysitting Katie and Ben. Ben was spending more time with me because Paula was drinking and smoking crack. Then I got a part-time job as a bartender at the Town and Country Inn from 3:00 p.m. to 2:00 a.m. I was working, getting everyone off to school, bowling three times a week, and sleeping maybe three hours a night. I tried not to go home or spend any time with my family. People at work thought that I was going through a personality change. I would go sit in a corner and not say anything. I started drinking again and smoking marijuana. Anything to escape reality."

"I just didn't care anymore," Becca said. Her eyes had taken on the chill of winter; her moods bounced between bliss and despair; and she moved like molasses on a wooden floor. "I think Chad began to see that something was wrong. I wasn't spending time with the girls. Paula stopped by the house to see how I was doing. When Paula saw Chad hit Dani in her face, Paula took the girls to her house and came to work and told me what happened. I just shook my head as if I didn't care and told her that Dani was his daughter. That was so unlike me," Becca added.

"The next day, I told Chad that I needed to check myself into the hospital. I was losing my mind. I remember packing some clothes and telling Amanda and Dani goodbye. I remember driving towards the hospital on a Saturday morning. Then, I remember waking up on Monday morning in a motel room. I don't know how I got there. Paula must have seen me that weekend. She had called Chad and told him that I was acting strange, and she thought that there was something wrong with me. He told her that I was supposed to be in the hospital. Chad began looking for me and found me at the motel. He took me home where I slept a lot and wouldn't talk with anyone." On the weekend prior to Dani's death, Chad continued to yell and scream at Becca, and wouldn't allow her to sleep. "I was exhausted and just wanted Chad to take Dani and leave," Becca said. "I felt a lot of hatred for Chad. I could feel it building inside." Chad followed Becca from one room to the other, like an unwanted shadow. It was Saturday, Sunday, then Monday, and finally Tuesday. I had asked Becca to describe what she remembered about that Tuesday morning.

Katie's mom dropped her by our house at 4:30 a.m. I told her to go climb in bed with Dani. I begged Chad to go to work so he wouldn't lose his new job. He left around 6:00 a.m. I let Katie and Dani sleep until 7:00 a.m. I got them up and took Katie to school. When Dani and I came home, Chad had returned. He just wouldn't leave me alone. Dani got out of the car and ran into the house and to her room. I went straight to the bathroom where I began drawing a bath for Dani. Chad followed me from one room to another. I can't remember what he said. His screams had become a blur. I went back to the bathroom and shut off the water. I started back to Dani's room to get her ready for her bath. Chad was still screaming. Then, I remember waking up on the floor in front of Dani's bedroom. I looked around and saw Dani lying on the floor. She didn't move. I thought she was dead. Chad was gone. I panicked and called one of my friends for help. She wasn't home. I grabbed Dani, carried her to the car, and raced to the emergency room. When I carried her inside, I was screaming and crying and telling them that Dani was dead. They told me that she was not dead and hooked her up to a monitor to show me that her heart was still beating. They called Chad at work and he told the nurses to ask me what happened. I told them that I didn't know.

As we sat at a table in the visit room, I couldn't help but wonder what happened on that Tuesday morning. While I gently pushed Becca to search her memory, I was concerned that what might surface could be harmful to her mental state. "Do you remember hitting Dani?" I asked.

"No. I don't remember doing anything to her."

"How do you know that you killed her?" I asked.

"Because they told me I did," Becca answered. "They said that I confessed to it."

"But you don't remember doing it? Is that right?"

"Yes," she said.

I couldn't help but wonder if Becca killed Dani. My mind kept telling me that it had to be Becca. Still, I had doubts. "Is it possible that Chad had something to do with it?" I asked.

"What do you mean?" Becca said.

"Well, he does have a history of violence. And you said that he had come back to the house and was there when you blacked out. Then he was gone when you later woke up. He could have been involved and then left and went to work. It's possible."

"I never thought about that," she said. She seemed to be puzzled as she searched her memory. "I don't think I want to know that," she said. "This is my life. I'm stuck in here. How would I feel if I found out that he did it and I couldn't do anything about it?"

"Have you talked to the psychologist about this?" I asked.

Looking somewhat disturbed, she said, "No, I don't think that I'll be doing that."

I moved the conversation back to that Tuesday morning. "What happened after you took Dani to the hospital?" I asked.

Because of Dani's injuries, she was flown to a hospital in Peoria, where they were better prepared to deal with severe head trauma. While Dani flew by helicopter, Kevin, Chad's friend, drove Chad and Becca to the Peoria hospital. During the one hour drive, Becca said that she pressed her head against the passenger window and heard the tires pound on the uneven highway. "Chad was talking to Kevin about other stuff. He didn't seem concerned about Dani. I couldn't understand it. Kevin seemed a lot more upset than Chad." When they arrived at the hospital, they were allowed to spend fifteen minutes with Dani every three hours. "I held her hands," Becca said. The only sounds were the steady beep of the heart monitor and the hissing sound from the oxygen tank. "When I wasn't with her, I sat in the lobby and rocked back and forth. And then, two days later, it was over. Dani was gone."

Silence followed. Becca wiped the tears from her eyes. "I'm sorry," I said. "Becca, if you admit that you killed Dani, I will not think any less of you. I know that you are a good person and couldn't have known what you were doing at that time. Did you kill Dani?"

"I don't know," Becca answered. "But if I did kill Dani, I got the wrong person. Chad's the person that I wanted to kill."

Little White Box

It was small, barely two or three inches in height, and was tucked inside a letter that Becca had written to me on November 16, 2006. It was a photograph of Dani when she was barely five. I knew it was coming. Becca wanted me to know Dani, and had said she would send me a photo. But its effect on me was more than I expected. Now, as I held the picture, I was still, as if time rode the current and I was left at the river's edge. She was so young, this little girl; so pretty, so pure, all of the things that little girls are known for. She seemed angelic, with her newly formed wings ready to fly. She had long blond hair, blue eyes, skin the color of river pearls, and she sat at a desk with both arms stretched out over an open book. The front of her pink dress had a drawing of Minnie Mouse, and her collar was etched in white lace. I was reminded of my granddaughters.

Here I was, expected to write about this little girl and the woman who was accused of taking her life. I imagined the three of us sitting at a round table in the visit room, Becca to my left and Dani to my right. Dani had a pad of paper and a stack of worn-down crayons, and would sometimes look our way, smiling and showing rows of baby teeth. In other moments, her smile disappeared and a spiritual serenity filled our space, a compassion I had seldom felt before. Although I will never experience Dani's physical presence – her flesh and bones will never join us in the visit room – her spirit sits with me as I choose each word.

In a letter, Becca shared her thoughts. "I think, in the back of my head, that I saved Dani from more sexual abuse, but then I took her life. How could I do that? To save her just to kill her." Becca had told me that the boyfriend of Dani's mother had sexually abused Dani and that was the reason she and Chad were granted full custody. She believed that a lifetime of sexual abuse was inevitable for Dani, had she lived, and wondered whether such a fate might be worse than death. Her statements indicated a need for some justification of Dani's death and her own incarceration. Mental illness had distorted her judgment, leaving her to cling to the flawed notion that Dani might be better off dead.

In this letter, Becca wrote about the Tuesday when Dani was taken to the OSF St. Francis Medical Center, a state-of-the-art children's hospital in Peoria, Illinois. The Children's Hospital of

Cherry Blossoms & Barren Plains

Illinois, as it was commonly called, was first established in 1877 by The Sisters of the Third Order of St. Francis, whose intentions were honorable: to show the love and care of a community that celebrated the gift of life. What began in a two story wooden framed house, grew into one of the largest medical centers in the country. Located in the historical section of Peoria, the modern structure covers several city blocks, and houses 731 beds with more than 5,000 employees and a medical staff of some 750 people. It has a level 1 trauma center and a helicopter transport program that carried Dani to the hospital that would surely save her life.

They were all sitting in a waiting room – Chad's family, Tammy's family, and Becca. The doctor, dressed in his pale-blue hospital scrubs, walked into the room and told them that there was significant swelling in Dani's brain. He explained that a severe head injury produces an additional amount of blood, which, in turn, increases the size of the brain; that barbiturates are sometimes used to induce a temporary coma, which reduces the metabolic rate of brain tissue, as well as the cerebral blood flow; and when successful, the blood vessels in the brain narrow, decreasing the size of the brain, and hence, the intra-cranial pressure. He was going to induce a coma; this was her only chance.

From the Streator ER to St. Francis, from her death to the wake and finally the funeral, and from the autopsy report to the detective's interrogation, a story began to unfold. It evolved slow and sure like a winter storm: gusts of wind blew up in the Rockies and crept across the Kansas plains into Missouri, and developed into a storm that hit this family in Illinois. Now, as the doctor left the waiting room, family members began to question how Dani had ended up on the bedroom floor. The family could not yet imagine what the detectives would later allege; maybe there had been neglect, or maybe someone shook Dani too hard. That's what they thought, nothing more.

"I remember everyone yelling at each other and looking for someone to blame. Chad's dad needed someone to blame, to have peace. I loved him and Chad's mom like my own parents. They could blame me. That was okay. I couldn't let them blame Chad. They knew what Chad was capable of and I didn't want it to be worse for Chad. Why? I don't know." I later asked Becca if she was implying that Chad was the one who had injured Dani. That was not her intent, she claimed. "They knew that Chad could be a violent man. I didn't want them to assume that he did it. That would have made it more difficult for them." While they sat in the waiting room, trying to sort through the doctor's latest comments, Tammy announced that she was pregnant and would have another baby to replace Dani if she died. "That's when I jumped across the table and nearly chocked the life out of Tammy," Becca said. "I think I could have killed her at that moment. Chad pulled me off." Becca's irritability and fits of rage had happened before, and were regarded as symptoms of bipolar disorder.

Becca ran out of the room, down the hallway, and up the spiral staircase to the roof's edge. Darkness had moved in. Passing cars looked like lightning bugs from a distance, while a north-westerly wind pushed the November temperature to the low forties. "I stood on the edge and looked down at the parking lot," Becca said. "Chad grabbed my arm. I think that God must have sent Chad to save me. For what? I don't know.

Time at St. Francis' was measured by the steady beep of Dani's heart monitor and the haunting back-and-forth movement of Becca as she sat in the waiting room. "I was so tired," Becca said. "No one knew that Chad and I had been fighting for days. I heard voices all around me but I didn't know where they were coming from." There were moments when Chad's father, still unaware of what Becca might have done, held Becca, and the two of them rocked together, trying to soothe each other's pain. But for the most part, Becca wrestled her misery in solitary silence, while she searched for understanding and reminisced on happier times. "Dani enjoyed the Dairy Queen. Hot dogs and a cheese sandwich were her favorites. She liked school, other children, and loved going to church. She called me mommy and thought that my children were her siblings." How ironic. The one who took her life was the one who loved her the most.

Early Wednesday morning, when Dani's death seemed certain, family members circled Dani for a hurried baptismal service. Two detectives pulled Becca aside and asked what had happened in her house the morning Dani was injured. "I couldn't answer them. I just remembered running the bath and going downstairs to wash a load of clothes that never got started. That's all I knew." A few hours later, the doctor came to the waiting room, asking to take Dani off of life support; there was nothing else they could do. Becca went to Dani's room, held her, and rocked back-and-forth. "I cried and told her how much I loved her. Two hours later we left with Chad's cousin who drove us back to Streator. Chad told me to stop crying. He was tired of hearing it. I turned and looked out the car window so he wouldn't see my tears continue to flow. We stayed at Chad's parents that night. I couldn't go back to our house."

Tammy and her half sister spent most of Thursday morning at Chad's parents, but when it came time to make funeral arrangements, Tammy had other things to do. Becca, Chad, and his family talked about how they needed to find a cemetery plot, pick out a casket, choose her clothes, find a minister, all of the things that proper planning required. "We needed just the right dress. We decided to use the dress that Dani wore at our wedding and the hair piece that she loved. She liked having long hair. Chad's mom made arrangements for the pastor at the Open Bible Church to speak at the funeral. This was the church where Dani went on our Wednesday bowling night."

Becca stayed at Chad's parents'. Chad spent the afternoon at Becca and Chad's house while detectives from the state crime lab looked for traces of blood, hair fibers, or pieces of human skin; anything that might tell them what happened on that Tuesday morning. "They went through everything," Becca said. "They ripped the house apart but they didn't find any blood or any kind of weapon. They even went through our cars. One detective later told me that Chad showed no remorse that his daughter was dead. Chad spent all of his time at the computer playing games while they tore the house apart. Maybe that was Chad's way of dealing with Dani's death. And then one of the detectives told me that Dani's head injuries were like she had been dropped out of a helicopter at sixty feet. I couldn't say anything. I just looked at him."

Another detective called Becca and said that he was waiting for the autopsy report, and that he would be out of town for a few days. He told her not to leave town and not to spend any time with her children. Except for Amanda, the other children were still in West Virginia with their grandparents. "I called Amanda and told her that we couldn't see each other. She cried and didn't understand. Then she asked about Dani's funeral. We made arrangements for her to come to the funeral home when I wasn't there. It was hard."

That night, while Chad's family was talking or watching television, Becca slipped out the back door and walked to her house. Since the roof incident at the hospital, the family had decided that Becca should not be left alone, and believed that she was in their bedroom upstairs. "I felt closed in and needed some fresh air to breathe. And I needed to pick up Dani's dress and hair piece that was packed away at my house."

Becca shuffled the three block walk to her house, like she was moving through mud. But when the front door opened, her feelings came alive. "I went to Dani's room and smelled her pillow, rubbed my fingers over her clothes, and held her dolls. I even sat in her closet with all of her shoes and stuff." Becca began to gather the things – the beanie baby collection, her favorite toys, and a necklace that her parents bought for Dani – that Dani treasured the most. Becca went down stairs and searched for the hair piece that was packed away, and then made her way up the stairs and down the hallway. There, standing in the doorway, was Dani. "She was real," Becca said. "Dani looked at me and told me that she loved me and that the truth will come out. Then I lost it. I ran out the door, dropped to my knees, and threw up on my front lawn. I ran all the way back to Chad's parents house. They were all mad because I left without telling them. But after they saw me crying and shaking, they didn't say anything. I ran up the stairs to where Chad was taking a shower. I told him what happened and that I had seen Dani. He slapped me and told me that she wasn't real, and that I was acting crazy. He told me not to tell anyone. So I never did. You're the first to know."

On Friday, Becca made a tape of songs which would be played at the funeral service; some songs were Dani's favorites, and others were one's that Amanda and Dani had enjoyed together. "I cried and tortured myself mentally as I put the tape together. Chad's dad still has the tape. He said that it reminded him of Dani and me." Becca and Chad's parents picked out the casket. There were several to choose from; some were rose colored, others were veneered in different shades of wood with ornamental handles – gold plated, nickel, and shinny chrome. They even chose a vault; Illinois law required it. A liner was mandatory, as well. The price of the liner determined how air-tight the seal would be, which, in turn, determined how long the body would be protected from water seepage. Finding a resting place was so painful, especially for one so young. When I asked about the casket and what it looked like, Becca said, "I don't remember the details. I just remember that it was small and white. It was like a little white box."

Becca's parents, Brent and Carolyn, traveled from West Virginia and arrived at Streator on Friday morning. "My dad was mad. He said that I was skinny and looked terrible. He went off on Chad for letting me get this way." When Becca was off her medications and in a manic state, she often stopped eating and sleeping, and lacked a center to her life. Her physical stature took on a more anorexia-like appearance, and her eyes looked empty. She was a Becca her parents had seen before.

Meanwhile, Aunt Marlene's sister, who worked at a local restaurant – a favorite among police officers who gathered for lunch, a cup of coffee, or maybe a piece of homemade pie – heard chatter between officers. It was not the serious talk that might jeopardize a case; it was more of the passing conversation made during a meal or after a deep pull from a cigarette. But the image of a dead five-year-old girl, caused words to stick in the air, waiting to be grabbed by someone sitting near. They supposed and theorized about what might have happened on the Tuesday morning that had escaped Becca's memory. Even today, Becca's memories are, at best, mere fragments or glimpses of a scene that has a big black hole in the middle, and awakens to an image of Becca opening her eyes and seeing Dani lying on the bedroom floor. As hard as she tries, the memories dart up and down, here and there, and evade her grasp like the illusive flight of a hummingbird. It was not idle talk at the restaurant that day. Marlene's sister called the family and said that Becca might need an attorney.

The wake was on Friday night. Family and friends filed through the funeral home, which looked more like an old house with plush carpet and creaky floors. "Me and Chad's parents pretty much planned everything. I fixed Dani's hair and put on the hair piece. I put the necklace and some of Dani's toys in the casket. It was hard but I did it. I couldn't believe all of the flowers." Flowers of different sizes and shapes flanked both sides of the casket, and Dani must have looked like she was nestled into a little white box in the middle of a flower garden. The presence of a butterfly or a tiny bird would have made the garden scene complete.

"The grief was heavy that night," said Raymond Rickert, the pastor at a church in Streator where Becca's parents had attended. Rickert said that Becca was distraught; not wailing or out of control, but very depressed and sad, as sad as one could imagine. When he tried to comfort Becca's mother, Carolyn, he was surprised by her response. "It's only going to get worse," Carolyn said. At the time, Rickert did not know the cause of Dani's death. He assumed Dani had fallen, that it was the result of some accident. Days later, when Becca signed her confession, he learned the extent of Carolyn's concerns.

Dani's death was different from most. When an elderly person died, family and friends celebrated his/her passing to a better place. But with someone so young, the pain settled hard. While there were the failed attempts to measure sadness by one's loss and the unfairness of it all, grief was abstract and impossible to define; how do you describe a broken heart? Dani's laughter was gone. Only the muffled sounds of whispers and the cries from mourners could be heard. And then the stares, the awful stares, and now at last, the suspicions as to what Becca might have done to Dani on that Tuesday morning. "There was a lot of fighting at the wake," Becca said. "Tammy's family wanted a share of the donations made to Dani. But the money was to be used for funeral expenses. Not to be split up among family members. Finally I told everyone to shut up. That someone we all loved had died. My mom and Chad's dad grabbed me and calmed me down but then they decided that I was right."

After the wake, Chad insisted on going to the local bar. "You would never have known by the way that Chad was carrying on that his daughter had just died. He was drinking and having a good time. I just sat in the corner and cried. Then Paul, one of Chad's friends, came to the bar looking for us. He came over and held me, and talked Chad into leaving the bar. After they dropped me at his parents' house, Chad and Paul went to our house where they spent the night."

Becca's memory of the Saturday funeral is spotty at best. Her mental illness, and the sadness of it all, had worn her down. "I was so numbed out," Becca said. "I was in a fog. I kept trying to hold myself together. I had to get through it." She remembers going to the funeral home and listening to Aunt Marlene sing a song that her aunt had written for Dani; she remembers how pretty Dani looked; and she remembers placing a rose on top of the casket as it was lowered into a deep dark hole. But she doesn't remember the cemetery. It must have been one of Streator's small-town cemeteries. Perhaps there were different sizes, shapes, and colors of granite, forming a field of carved stone, each with a name tag marking its home. Only the grass was green, while the trees were dormant. It was late November, too early for a hard freeze, so the backhoe would have had an easy dig. The grave was some six feet ten inches long by two feet seven inches wide, and dug to a depth of four feet six inches, and a large mound of black dirt, partially covered by fake green grass, was piled to one side. Family

Cherry Blossoms & Barren Plains

members sat in wooden folding chairs and faced the closed casket, while the pastor read words from an open book. First friends, and then family, walked away. Becca, the last to leave, stood and leaned forward, and dropped a red rose on the little white box.

Larry L Franklin

Broken Mind

> *Dani Lynn Bivens died on November, 18, 1998 at OSF Saint Francis Medical Center in Peoria of brain hemorrhaging caused by shaking, multiple blows to the head, and a "massive" skull fracture, Peoria pathologist Violetter Hinlica said. The pathologist also testified that the severe head injuries suffered by the victim "could only have been inflicted by another human being."*
> *Peoria Journal Star, July 30, 1999*

Dani's death changed the lives of so many. While the taking of a child's life cried out for a reason, logic was smothered by bellows for justice and a yearning for revenge; understanding gave way to quick, simplistic conclusions. How could Becca have killed a little girl whom she loved as her own? To search for answers, we must question the concept of free will, that everyone who commits a violent act is capable of making a choice between right and wrong. We must calm the cries for full accountability, that everyone be held accountable for their actions. This requires an open mind, an open heart, and the desire to understand the mentally ill and to explore the mysteries of the human brain.

The brain, some three pounds of gray matter suspended in cerebrospinal fluid, has over one-hundred billion nerve cells called neurons. Each neuron, just a tiny fraction of an inch and shaped like the root ball of a recently planted tree, has three parts: the cell body, the dendrites, and the axon. The nucleus of the cell body produces a substance needed for cell growth and maintenance. The tiny, hair like dendrites connect to one end of the cell body and receive signals from other neurons. The axon, which looks like the tip of a freshly picked carrot, is a single tube-like structure connected to the bottom end of the cell body. More hair-like fibers, called terminals, are connected to the axon and reach out, but don't quite touch the neighboring neurons. When information is transferred from one neuron to another, the gap between the terminals and nearby neurons is filled by chemical substances called neurotransmitters, which fire across the space, sending signals to other neurons. At times, brain activity might resemble a well-lit midway at a county fair, with hundreds of rides and booths operating simultaneously.

Cherry Blossoms & Barren Plains

Communication between and among neurons dictates such things as how we walk, how we raise an arm or sit on a stool, how we order a cup of coffee, and how our behavior is controlled. Messages are transported by those neurotransmitters that control and create signals that jump between neurons, like tiny sparks of electricity. There are some 50 different neurotransmitters in the brain. Four of the more common ones connected with emotional disorders are dopamine, serotonin, norepinephrine, and gamma-aminobutyric acid. Too much or too little of these neurotransmitters may contribute to schizophrenia, depression, bipolar disorder, and other emotional conditions. When neurotransmitters do not function properly, the client, like Becca, is said to have a "chemical imbalance."

Clinical psychologist Joseph M. Carver uses the metaphor of the fluid levels in an automobile to illustrate how neurotransmitters work in the human brain. Imagine an automobile and how it has a variety of fluids, from engine oil, to transmission fluid, to brake fluid, and a coolant for proper temperature control. All fluids must be at an acceptable level if the automobile is to run smoothly. Certain fluid levels, like engine oil and transmission fluid, can be checked with a dip stick, while others are gauged by marked indicators. In the human body, a simple blood test checks a host of conditions, like sugar and protein levels, nutrients, electrolytes, minerals, and whether the cholesterol level is too high. Patients with elevated cholesterol are told to take prescribed medications and to make adjustments in their life styles. While research science uses an advanced imaging technique called Positron Emission Tomography (PET) Scans to identify certain neurotransmitters, most mental health professionals measure levels of neurotransmitters the old-fashioned way: an interview where a medical history is taken and the client is questioned for clues to identify his or her thought process, sexual interest, appetite, sleep patterns, current and changing moods, beliefs and speech patterns. The professional then determines whether the client is in need of medication, psychological counseling, or both.

A knowledge of neurotransmitters is needed to understand the range of psychiatric conditions and to prescribe the proper medication. Although the neurotransmitter dopamine is commonly associated with Parkinson's disease, a motor-control disorder, it can influence the thinking part of the brain as well. Low levels of dopamine impede the client's ability to concentrate and to stay on task. With higher levels of dopamine, the client becomes more centered, but if the levels are too elevated, the client is excited, more suspicious, and even paranoid. Serotonin is like the engine oil that keeps the auto running smoothly. It regulates many emotions that can cause the client to experience a span of feelings from bliss to despair. Psychologists believe that too little serotonin can lead to severe depression, while too much serotonin can lead to feelings of elation and even to a life-threatening condition called serotonin syndrome. Norepinephrine acts like an adrenaline that is unleashed in the brain, causing a "fight or flight" response. High levels of norepinephrine may create anxiety and panic attacks. Low levels leave a stagnant state of mind; medium levels work like a stimulant and promote a pleasurable sensation, similar to the high from a snort of cocaine.

The neurotransmitter GABA, gamma-aminobutyric acid, is often mentioned in the treatment of Bipolar Disorder, the mental illness that commandeered Becca's brain. GABA restricts the links between neurons by decreasing the ability of neurotransmitters to communicate. If not controlled, neurotransmitters such as dopamine, serotonin and norepinephrine, can wreak havoc within the brain circuits that control emotion and anxiety. While too little GABA produces a manic state that allows neurotransmitters to run rampant and fan anxiety like a wildfire, high levels of GABA lead to depression. Controlling proper levels of GABA is essential in the treatment of Bipolar Disorder. A patient in a manic state with low levels of GABA is commonly treated with lithium. A patient in a depressed state with high levels of GABA and low serotonin is often treated with lithium and SSRIs, Selective Serotonin Reuptake Inhibitors.

The purpose of medication is to control the level of neurotransmitters that flow from one neuron to another. This is done by *tricking* the neurons into changing their actions based on the assumption that they have received an increased or decreased level of neurotransmitters. Some medications act like chameleons. They imitate the neurotransmitter, triggering a response as though the original neurotransmitter were present, while other medications block the neurotransmitter from being absorbed by the surrounding neurons. This is known as "blocking the reuptake." Reuptake inhibitors block the reabsorption/reuptake of serotonin or norepinephrine and thus make more neurotransmitters available. Certain medications force the release of the neurotransmitter, causing an exaggerated effect, while some medications increase neurotransmitters known to slow down or reduce the production of other neurotransmitters. Other medications block the release of neurotransmitters completely.

At 6:30 each evening, when most people sit at their dinner table or watch the national news, Becca stands in the med line at the Dwight Correctional Center. Inmates are handed a small white paper cup filled with prescribed medications. Becca's cup holds Lithium, a small silvery white-gray pill, and Paxil, one more oval shaped and pink in color. Each pill is followed by a sip of water, a noticeable swallow, and an open mouth, just so the guard can make certain that no pills are stored for later use. Although pharmacology – the science of drugs – has made rapid strides since the middle of the twentieth century, it lacks the precision of a surgical knife, where deep cuts can remove a cancerous tumor or mend an unwanted embolism. Pharmacology is not an exact science.

According to Robert M. Julien in *A Primer of Drug Action*, psychoactive drugs alter mood, thought process, or behavior, and are used to manage neuropsychological illness. We learn that "drugs are effective treatment for disease, that drug dosage and drug responsiveness are related, that drugs act at specific sites of action, that potency and efficacy are different, and that specific drug receptors can be characterized." The process, from the drug's absorption, to distribution, to metabolism, and, finally, to its elimination, is called pharmacokinetics. The time of onset and the drug's duration determines the course of action: the drug, the optimal dosages and dose intervals, and the therapeutic drug level needed to accomplish the desired result.

The pea-sized pill moves through the body like a mouse through a maze. First, the pill is absorbed in the stomach, penetrates the lining of the intestines and races through the blood stream to its intended target. Every minute the heart pumps the body's entire volume of blood throughout the circulatory system. To achieve the intended affect, psychoactive drugs must bind to and interact with receptors located on the surface of certain neurons in the brain. This interaction changes the functional properties of that neuron, and thus, helps create the preferred behavior. At any given time, only a small portion of the medication is attached to the attended receptor in the brain. The rest of the drug languishes in other parts of the body where it may cause unpleasant side effects. Eventually the drug is metabolized by the liver and excreted by the kidneys. The process is repeated until the desired level and duration of the drug is reached, and a steady state is maintained.

Although an accepted form of treatment by the American Psychiatric Association and modern medicine, Pharmacology is not without its critics. The internet carries stories about the side-effects of psychoactive drugs and how they can lead to suicide, a loss of identity, or a dysfunctional mind at best. Manufacturers of antidepressants are now required to post a warning that when the drugs are given to minors, there is an increased risk of suicide. Peter R. Breggin, author of *Toxic Psychiatry: Why Therapy, Empathy, and Love Must Replace the Drugs, Electroshock and Biochemical Theories of the "New Psychiatry,"* hammers away at the current state of psychiatric care, claiming that the use of drugs destroy one's memory and cognitive abilities. Most recently, we have heard the criticism of famous actors, John Travolta and Tom Cruise, who espouse the teachings of Scientology, that psychoactive drugs can destroy the human mind. Travolta went so far as to blame the recent school shootings of Columbine and Virginia Tech on the perpetrators use of psychoactive drugs. L. Ron Hubbard, founder of Scientology, encourages his followers to think in terms of the human brain as being divided into two sections: the reactive brain and the analytical brain. The reactive brain is the part that holds the negative memories that lead to irrational behavior and needs only to be cleared to experience true mental health.

To put an unknown substance into your body requires a measure of faith, a degree of desperation, and possibly, a healthy dose of fear. Now, some ten years after Dani's death, Becca's primary motivation is fear. The memory that she might have killed Dani hounds her like a shadow, and is a reminder of what could happen if she doesn't take her medications.

Becca first took Lithium in late 1993, stopped taking the drug in 1996, and restarted in late 1998. It continues to be the drug of choice for the treatment of bipolar disorder. When taken orally, a daily dosage reaches peak levels in three hours and is completely absorbed within eight hours, and accumulates slowly over two weeks before reaching a steady state Julien reports a study citing a success rate of eighty-eight per cent in the treatment of manic episodes. In a similar study, twenty-eight per cent of participants discontinued the use of Lithium; thirty-eight per cent continued the medication but experienced further episodic recurrences; and twenty-three per cent reported no further problems. Suicide attempts declined by seventy-seven per cent. But when treatment was discontinued, the suicide rate increased fourteen fold.

A Serotonin-Specific Reuptake Inhibitor (SSRI) is often used in combination with lithium, and may be effective in treating depression. Becca takes the SSRI Paxil. The medications take away the highs and drop the lows, and leave her somewhere in between. Perhaps she looks in the mirror and is puzzled by what she sees: a cicada whose body has slipped away and left its shell. "I'm a different person," she says. "I don't feel the same."

"Can you help me look inside your head?" I once asked, as we sat in the visit room. "Tell me what it's like to be bipolar?"

Without hesitation, Becca told me to go see the movie *Mr. Jones*. "When I first saw the movie, I broke down and cried. I told my husband that this is what it is like to be bipolar. That's the way it is. Exactly."

Mr. Jones is a movie released in 1993 where Richard Gere plays a man who is suffering from bipolar disorder. We see the inner intoxication that he sometimes feels, and the debilitating depression, when he is locked up in a mental hospital and drugged into a stupor. We see him plead with his psychiatrist that he just wants to be himself, that his mania is quite normal, and that drugs alter who he is.

Becca's mental illness was compounded by the violence unloaded on her – the busted face, the broken nose, the loaded words, the knife in the back of her hand – that stirred up the chemical imbalance in her brain, causing neurotransmitters to pop and crackle like bacon on a hot grill. She didn't stand a chance for a normal life. Violence was the constant agitator that contributed to her mental illness; craziness was her reality. Was her path self inflicted; was she somehow condemned at birth with DNA that drove her like a guided missile; or was she the recipient of repeated trauma that twisted and broke her mind?

The debate between nature and nurture persists. Nature tattoos us with a genetic makeup, DNA, that determines who we are in many fundamental ways. Nurture is a product of what we see, hear, smell, and touch, and the countless life experiences that mold our core. Developmental biology tells us that we are a combination of the two. From the beginning, we are organisms with a genetic blueprint that continually interacts with our environments, causing change to occur as we move from conception, to childhood, to adulthood, and finally to death. In her book *The Biology of*

Violence, Debra Niehoff says, "Even the most unrepentant assailants, the most cold-blooded murderers, the most sadistic of serial killers, were once infants. There was a time when they could barely hold a rattle, much less a gun; when they smiled for Christmas portraits and giggled at peek-a-boo; when they were afraid of fireworks, needed help to feed themselves, and wore shoes no bigger than ring boxes. What happened? What inner or outer factor – parents, schools, genes, morals, abuse, television, neglect, stress, attention deficits, self-esteem, temperament – has the power to transform innocence into violence? The answer provided by modern neuroscience is 'all of the above.'"

Niehoff considers behavior to be a dialogue, a communication "between past and present, experience and physiology." Instead of looking only to our genetic makeup as the cause of behavior, the action that sets the neurobiological process in motion is equally important. Our brain is a historian that records each life experience which ultimately influences the flow of neurotransmitters between neurons. Michael Zigmond, at the University of Pittsburgh, conducted a study concerning the effects that repeated stress has on one of the neurotransmitters, norepinephrine. Zigmond separated rats into two groups; group one was confined to a cold room for three weeks, while group two was housed in a low-stress, temperature-controlled environment. Both groups were subsequently given a mild electric shock. Group one, the previously stressed rats, recorded more than a two-and-a-half times greater surge of norepinephrine, which, in turn, created an elevated "fight or fright" response.

Humans show similar responsive behaviors. Clients suffering from Post Traumatic Stress Disorder have significantly higher urinary levels of norepinephrine than clients without the disorder. Repeated trauma in humans changes the levels of norepinephrine, and in turn, changes their behavior. There can be little doubt that violence in Becca's life aggravated her mental illness. Many people in her world felt emotions held in bay by a hair trigger, ready to fire at the slightest irritant. They lacked good judgment and the ability to reason. Life was a series of knee-jerk reactions, a continuous circle where bad genes, bad environment, and bad chemistry fed on each other, and grew into an octopus-like creature, the one that I imagined.

Cherry Blossoms & Barren Plains

Confession

On or about November 17, 1998 in LaSalle County, Illinois, Rebecca S. Bivens, Defendant, committed the offense of First Degree Murder in that the said Defendant, without lawful justification, punched Dani Bivens, age five, in the face and head with her fist, slapped Dani Bivens across both sides of her head, placed both hands on the shoulders of Dani Bivens and shook Dani Bivens, picked Dani Bivens up and threw Dani Bivens across a room causing Dani Bivens to strike her head on a wooden arm rest of a love seat, and slammed the head of Dani Bivens on a coffee table, all with such force as to fracture the skull of Dani Bivens, knowing such acts created a strong probability of death or great bodily harm to Dani Bivens, thereby causing the death of Dani Bivens, in violation of Section 5/9-1(a)(2) Chapter 720, Illinois Compiled Statutes. Charges made by the State of Illinois against Rebecca S. Bivens.

It was a Sunday afternoon, five days after the death of Dani Bivens, when the police told Chad and Becca to come to the police station; some questions needed to be answered. At 5:00 p.m. Chad and Becca rode in their 1992 Blue Ford Escort to the Streator Police Station; it was a short drive, maybe twenty minutes at most. There was no conversation, no radio, just the sound of rolling tires on a blacktop road, and the hissing of air working its way around the window edge. Becca gazed out the front window, and wrestled the kind of worry that hits deep in your stomach and locks up your throat, making it difficult to speak.

Rigid and stone-faced, she asked, "Are they going to arrest me?"
"Probably," Chad said.

She knew that someone had to take the blame for Dani's death. "Even if I didn't do it," Becca later said, "I allowed it to happen. I was responsible."

I remember my first conversation with Becca at the Dwight Correctional Center. "You can ask me anything you want," Becca had said. "I have nothing to hide. I killed my five-year-old step-daughter but I don't remember doing it."

Months later, it dawned on me to ask the most logical question. "If you can't remember killing Dani, how do you know that you did it?"

My question surprised her. For an instant, her mind seemed to ponder the possibility that she might not have killed Dani. But then she jumped back to her programmed ways: "Because they told me I did." Were her blocked memories characteristic of a faulty mind, or evidence of a miraculous brain that sought to protect her from trauma? Much has been written about the phenomenal abilities of the human brain to filter emotional experiences, to bury what we cannot bear to know. But lost memories can rip a chunk from your soul. There's no history; there's no footprints in the snow.

Becca had a history of lost memory, sometimes called a dissociative fugue disorder, where her mind, for just a moment, a few hours, days, or sometimes more, drifted from reality. In 1993, Becca, at age 26, found herself in a small downtown apartment in Princeton, Illinois, with little memory of the previous six months. Working in a local bar and living in an upstairs apartment are all that she recalls. Becca was treated at Ottawa Community Hospital by Dr. Barr with a diagnosis of Bipolar Disorder, Borderline Personality Disorder, and Codependency. From 1995 to 1998, Becca suffered "blackouts" in her manic states. Her latest episode had been the weekend of November 7, 1998, when she found herself in a motel room in Streator, Illinois. Three or four days slid somewhere beneath her retrievable memories. The fact that she does not remember how Dani died is no surprise. It speaks directly to any suspicion of "convenient" memory lapse. Rather, it is consistent with a pattern that pre-dates Dani's death by a number of years.

While Chad talked with the police, Becca sat in seclusion and studied her thoughts. Images of Dani alive popped into her mind, a constant reminder that Dani was now dead. When it came her turn, Becca walked into the interrogation room, a small, rectangular space sparsely filled with sterile office furniture. Her mind was in disarray; she was mentally ill, a victim of domestic violence, and her five-year-old step-daughter had been killed. Becca's ability to reason had been diminished.

Becca's memories of the interrogation were sparse and dark, a mental forest burn. She remembers two police officers who were later joined by someone from the Department of Children and Family Services. She remembers asking for Chad and then, an attorney. But each time, Becca claims that the police told her that if she wasn't guilty she wouldn't need anyone. "They asked me to take a lie detector test. I should have taken it. I've always wondered what it would have said." Even today, some nine years after Dani's death, Becca would welcome a polygraph, if for no other reason than to know whatever truth might be buried in her own unconscious.

Although Becca told the police that she didn't remember what happened on that Tuesday morning, they began to speculate about what might have occurred. They referred to the pathologist's report and pictures of Dani's battered head, and suggested that Becca might have hit Dani, or maybe she threw her across the room, or shook her in a fit of rage. They thought perhaps that Becca didn't like Dani and wanted to get rid of her. What came out of the lengthy interrogation was a signed confession that laid out a methodical procedure, showing how Becca ended Dani's life. Becca slammed her fist into the side of Dani's face, slapped both sides of her head, threw her across the room, causing her head to strike the wooden arm rest of a love seat, and, finally, slammed Dani's head on the top of a coffee table. It was a confession she doesn't remember and one that she rejects. "That confession was not me," Becca said. "There's no way on earth I would have done something like that to Dani. I loved her."

Becca later said that she didn't know that she had signed a confession until her defense attorney met with her several weeks after her arraignment. "When he asked me about my confession, I said what confession? He told me that I had signed one and showed me a copy. I don't know how I could have signed such a thing." Although the Streator Police Department had the technology to do an audio or video recording of Becca's interrogation, none was done. We are left to wonder about Becca's state of mind and what went on behind those closed doors. We have only the explanation of the police and the memories of a confused woman.

Whether Becca was guilty or not, her mental state at the time of her interrogation raises the possibility of a false confession. John E. Reid, author of *Criminal Interrogation and Confession*, defines coerced internalized confessions as, "Confessions that are allegedly false and occur when the investigator successfully convinces an innocent suspect that he/she is guilty of a crime he/she does not remember committing." According to Reid, this accounts for 21 percent of false confessions.

Psychiatrist Terence W. Campbell says, "Coerced internalized confessions occur when anxious, confused suspects feel overwhelmed by very suggestive interrogation tactics. In particular, interrogators typically offer suspects a rationale as to how they could have committed the crime, and then forgotten it."

With a signed confession in hand, the detectives moved Becca to a holding cell, a three-sided concrete-walled room with a screen of metal bars in front. Hours later, she was transferred by a Streator police car to the LaSalle County Jail in Ottawa, where she was allowed to call her mother and Aunt Marlene. "When I told them what had happened," Becca said, "they both cried. I called Chad but he wasn't home." Becca said that she didn't sleep that night; she just sat in her cell and rocked back and forth. Early the next morning, when most people were going to work or finishing their second cup of coffee, Becca was led to the LaSalle County Courthouse and arraigned for first degree murder with a two million dollar bond. The emotional crescendo had peaked and now, Becca was broken. "I lost it," Becca said. "They took me to the Ottawa hospital and admitted me to the mental ward. The next thing that I remember was waking up on Saturday morning. I had lost Tuesday, Wednesday, Thursday, and Friday."

***

April 23, 2007, some seven days after the nation's largest killing spree, the American people reeled from the murders at Virginia Tech, where Cho Seung-Hui single-handedly shot to death thirty-two fellow university students. The air waves were filled with the tragedies of young lives cut short, and Cho's troubled past. People looked for an easy answer, a single clue that explained how a person could slip into a fit of rage.

Decades ago, people understood less about criminal acts and mental illness. The reasons were clear: the killer did it and should be put to death or locked away. End of story. Today, David Brooks, a conservative columnist with *The New York Times*, writes about the nation's struggle to find a deeper understanding of what makes a killer.

"In short," Brooks writes, "the killings at Virginia Tech happen at a moment when we are renegotiating what you might call the Morality Line, the spot where background forces stop and individual choice – and individual responsibility – begins. The killings happen at a moment when the people who explain behavior by talking about biology, chemistry and social science are assertive and on the march, while the people who explain behavior by talking about individual character are confused and losing ground. And it's true. We're never going back. We're not going to put our knowledge of brain chemistry or evolutionary psychology back in the bottle. It would be madness to think Cho Seung-Hui could have been saved from his demons with better sermons."

The people of Streator wanted swift justice and to be left with a distant memory. They preferred the single melody that mirrored their preconceived ideas of what went wrong. But the facts mimic the complexities of a Mozart symphony, where harmony plays a role, secondary themes abound, counterpoint adds intrigue, and crescendos and decrescendos are peppered with staccatos and motifs, all strung together in separate movements that evolve into a single work.

For some, particularly the religious right, the idea that behavior is beyond our control is unthinkable. After all, free will is the glue that holds society to a moral standard that allows us to make conscious choices between right and wrong. The free will position is alive and well in our criminal system, as evidenced by the recent addition of adult sentences for juveniles, and the three strikes and you're out clause in the criminal code. Both laws are built upon the assumption that everyone has free will and should be held accountable for their actions. Even the insanity plea is seldom used in its previous form, and seems to be replaced by a plea of guilty, but insane.

The other extreme is determinism: human behavior is governed by causal laws, and can be explained by the careful examination of biological, psychological, and sociological characteristics. The idea that a criminal act is not a conscious choice removes blame and ultimately, the rationale for punishment. Instead, perpetrators might receive institutionalized medical treatment for their actions. This idea has little traction today.

American society is moving slowly towards soft determinism, a more moderate position somewhere between free will and absolute determinism. Proponents of soft determinism believe that human beings control a significant portion of their behavior, even though they are limited in their choices. If a person is about to commit a violent act, is the decision based on the same criteria as you or I would employ? Would a person who has been subjected to repeated trauma, or one who is a victim of domestic violence, or one who is mentally ill, have the same database to refer to when making decisions? Each person, controlled by genes and the effects of individual environments, responds uniquely to a given situation. Add severe mental illness to the formula and free will becomes less of a factor; possibly, it becomes nonexistent. Imagine, if you can, how Becca, someone diagnosed and treated for mental illness, a victim of domestic violence, and someone who suffered from extended blackouts, could control her behavior by a simple act of free will. It seems unlikely.

According to neuroscientist Niehoff, "The days of nature versus nurture are over... Our genes do affect the likelihood of violence. And so does our mature brain chemistry. And so does our environment, as well as the nurturing we get as children and the social life we have with our peers." And so does mental illness. Behavioral change is an ongoing process, and has a degree of flexibility. Behavior can be changed or, better yet, steered in the right direction through the use of pharmacology, talk therapy, and a changed environment. Like a metal spring, the human brain is somewhat elastic and can be reshaped. But if the spring has been stretched beyond recognition, or if it is allowed to maintain an irregular shape for too many years, the spring can be beyond repair.

***

Dr. Chuprevich, psychiatrist at the Ottawa Hospital, argued that Becca should stay in the mental ward and should not go back to jail. But Chuprevich's request was denied and Becca was returned to the LaSalle County Jail. "Things were confusing," Becca said. "The medicine they had me on kept me doped up really good. I was in my own little world, trying to cut my wrists with whatever I could get my hands on. None of the women prisoners wanted to be my roommate because I was a murderer. That broke my heart. They were all reading the stories about me in the Ottawa newspaper. How I had killed a little five-year-old girl. They called me baby killer." Becca said that Chad came to see her one time during her incarceration in the county jail. He was busy running around with other women and forging her social security checks. After she made several attempts to call Chad, the guards told her that Chad was in jail for taking a baseball bat to some girl's boyfriend.

On December 21, 1998, the defense attorney, Daniel J. Bute, sent Becca to a psychiatrist, Robert E. Chapman, in Bloomington, Illinois to determine whether she was fit to stand trial, and to determine her sanity at the time of the offense. The standard of fitness refers to 725 ILCS 5/104-10: "A defendant is unfit if because of his/her mental or physical condition he/she is unable to understand the nature and purpose of the proceedings against he/she or to assist in his/her defense." Insanity is defined by 720 ILCS 5/6-2: "A person is not criminally responsible for conduct if at the time of such conduct as a result of mental disease or defect he/she lacks substantial capacity to appreciate the criminality of his/her conduct."

Becca told Chapman, that since Chuprevich had placed her on medication on November 25th, she was "feeling 100 percent better," but admitted to "having good days and bad days." Each time, over the past several years, when Becca had been treated with medications, she gained some level of sanity. So why not take the medications? Why go for months and even years, avoiding the very thing that offered you hope? That must be the question most people ask who look from a distance. But from the inside, it's a different story. E. Fuller Torrey and Michael B. Knable, authors of <u>Surviving Manic Depression: A Manual on Bipolar Disorder for Patients, Families, and Providers</u>, say that "approximately half of the individuals stop taking their medication during a one-year period; another study found that half discontinued their medication over a two-year period." Torrey and Knable attribute medication noncompliance to the seduction of mania, lack of awareness of illness, side effects of medication, denial of illness, depression, delusions, cognitive deficits, fears of becoming dependent, and poor doctor-patient relationship.

For Becca, the reasons for noncompliance are many. But the one that stood out was the one she repeated the most: "When I was off my medication, I could handle the physical abuse from the men in my life. I could take anything they dished out." She added how prison would be a breeze if she was off her medication. "I wouldn't feel anything," she claimed.

Mania was her seducer, the gigolo, the lady's man, that pulled Becca into its trap. When you're in a manic state, life can be as good as it gets. How do you trade paradise for a regiment of medications that can be intolerable? Hand tremors, nausea, diarrhea, weight gain, hair loss, decreased coordination, irregular heart rhythms, decrease in sexual desire, and even the possibility of liver and kidney failure are potential side effects.

Becca's manic state sometimes left her with feelings of irritability and anger, followed by a deep depression, and a incoherent mental process that made her incapable of logic and rational thought. She sometimes asked for help when her manic highs dropped to her can't-move depressions. It wasn't enough for family and friends to say that Becca was just acting a little strange. They needed a better understanding of severe mental illness, while Becca needed a regimen of medication, talk therapy, and a changed environment.

Torrey believes that people with severe mental illness – schizophrenia and manic depressive illness – sometimes need mandatory assisted treatment. For whatever reason, the mentally ill can fail to realize that medication might be their only bridge to sanity. Until the drugs kick in, affected individuals lack the comprehension skills to determine whether or not they need help. Torrey and Knable refer to a study of twenty-seven individuals who were forced to take medications for a year. They were asked to reflect on the merits of such treatment. Nine were positive, three were negative, nine expressed mixed views, and six said that they had no feelings at all. In another study of thirty individuals who had been forced to take medications, they were asked for their opinions after being discharged. Eighteen were positive, nine were negative, and three were unsure.

Any mention of mandatory treatment rallies proponents for civil liberties. They think about days gone by when mental hospitals housed patients against their will, when no viable treatment plan was in place. The American Civil Liberties Union and the Bazelon Center for Mental Health Law in Washington, D.C. have vigorously opposed laws supporting mandatory treatment and have obtained court rulings in some states that make treatment impossible. How many people like Becca will end up homeless, incarcerated, commit suicide, or take someone's life, because they lacked proper care?

Becca told Chapman about imaginary voices that she had heard for the past seventeen years. In her depression stage, the voices said "You are no good." In her manic stage, the voices urged her to hurt others and to hurt herself. "The voices in my head are like continuous thoughts. My brain never shuts off."

Becca recalled the lost weekend on November 7th when she blacked out for days, not having a clue as to what she had done. She had no sleep the weekend prior to November 17th, and maybe forty-five minutes of sleep on November 16th. "My brain was going, going, racing, jumping as it did when I was in a manic state. I wrote things down on paper. It didn't make sense. I wrote it down so it wouldn't hurt. It was a release for me." In a discussion between Chad and Chapman, Chad said that Becca's altered mental state began toward the end of October 1998. She became more irritable. They were working different hours and didn't get to see much of each other, but he did observe her sitting for long hours before the television, writing down things she heard or anything that came to her mind.

Chapman administered a competency exam and asked Becca to define the following.

> **Defense Attorney:** "Dan Bute. He is the public defender and acts as my lawyer and defends me."
> **State's Attorney:** "To prosecute me."
> **Judge:** "A man to find you guilty or not."
> **Jury:** "People who find you guilty or not."
> **How many persons in a jury:** "I don't know."
> **Witness:** "Somebody that sees something and tells what they saw."
> **Could you call a witness:** "I guess so."
> **Plea bargain:** "When the state's attorney makes an offer and if we take it, that is a plea agreement."
> **What would she do if heard state's witness lie:** "Nothing."
> **Charge:** "First Degree Murder. I was charged with manslaughter and then it went to First Degree Murder."
> **Consequences if found guilty:** "Twenty years to the death penalty."

Chapman's personal evaluation determined no evidence of psychotic symptoms, hallucinations, or delusions. In addition, the results from The Minnesota Multiphasic Personality Inventory-2, (MMPI), a 567 true/false psychodiagnostic test designed to help identify personal, social, and behavior problems in psychiatric patients, were invalid, because of an excessive number of false answers. No reason was given for the errors. Initially, I surmised that Becca was unable to stay focused for such a lengthy test, or perhaps she was confused. I later asked Becca about the MMPI-2 examination and why she had so many false answers. She didn't remember the test or the meeting with Chapman. When asked about the number of false answers at Becca's trial, Chapman said that it was not an indication that Becca lied when taking the examination. It merely showed that there were an excessive number of false answers.

Becca had a way of "zoning out" or dissociating from traumatic events that were too overwhelming for her conscious mind to accept. We've all heard stories where individuals were raped or suffered through equally traumatic events, and had no recollection of the trauma. Although the event caused emotional damage, it was repressed. Becca could talk with someone, and at the same time, her mind would drift elsewhere, leaving her with no recollection of the conversation. Often times, at the Dwight Correctional Center, fellow inmates have to remind Becca to "come back. Where are you?" I have seen Becca's mind drift away. Her eyes look past me and her attention disappears, and I repeat her name until she returns. Psychologists call it dissociation, a defensive mechanism employed in response to severe trauma. For Becca, her dissociative abilities were so strong and so often used, that she developed what is called a dissociative disorder. When she took the MMPI-2 examination, she went through the motions, most likely marking a host of false answers, then effectively forgetting the event had occurred.

"It is my opinion," Chapman wrote, "given with a reasonable degree of medical and psychiatric certainty, based on the information available to me and examination of Rebecca Sue Bivens, that she currently suffers no mental condition that renders her unable to understand the nature and purpose of the proceedings against her or to assist in her defense."

"It is my opinion that her current psycho tropic medicines – Klonopin, Zoloft, Zyprexa, Cogentin, and Trazondone, do not produce a medication effect, and are not expected to significantly alter her level of awareness, alertness, and capacity to attend, participate, and contribute to the trial process." (In June of 1999, when Becca's mental condition had declined, Chapman's opinion had changed. He believed that Becca was unable to understand the nature and purpose of the trial, and unable to assist in her defense.)

"It is further my opinion," Chapman wrote, "that on or about 17 November 1998 at the time of her conduct for which she is charged, Rebecca Sue Bivens suffered the mental disease of mania, acute state, and as a result of the symptoms thereof, it caused her to lack substantial capacity to appreciate the criminality of her conduct."

Raymond Rickert, a local minister, visited Becca on several occasions while she was incarcerated at the LaSalle County Jail. "Sometimes he would visit me three times a week," Becca said. Now, some nine years later, Rickert is retired but still makes an occasional trip to visit Becca at the Dwight Correctional Center. My telephone conversations with Rickert gave me the impression that he is a kind, gentle man who chooses his words carefully, and who believes that "not guilty by reason of insanity" would have been the proper verdict.

He described Becca's early days at the LaSalle County Jail. "Her mind was blurry," Rickert said. "At first she said that something terrible had happened to Dani. Days later, it was changed to the possibility that she had done something to Dani, and finally, to the realization that she had indeed done something very bad. But she never remembered what happened." I do not know if Becca's move toward an acknowledgment of her participation was due to the possibility that she remembered killing Dani, or if she finally accepted, without knowing, what the state was saying: that she had killed Dani. Rickert admitted to never asking Becca about her mental illness, her abusive past, or what happened on the Tuesday morning that Dani was injured. He was surprised when I told him that Chad might have been at the house when Becca blacked out and later awoke next to Dani on the bedroom floor. To the best of his recollection, no one had heard that story.

When I asked Rickert if their conversations were more of a spiritual nature, he said that in the beginning they were not. "I tried to help her reach a position where she could be more accepting of what happened, and to become more prepared for the trial that lay ahead." At first, Becca wanted to know what to expect, what were her options, and how much time she might serve. She was consumed by her dilemma. Over time, he explained, Becca became more stable and more accepting of her situation. She wanted to move forward. When Becca finally reached some level of stability, Rickert suggested that she ask herself, and then God, for forgiveness.

LaSalle County Jail

The LaSalle County Jail – aged, weather beaten, and too small to hold the growing number of inmates – showed the effects of time. Located in the center of Ottawa, Illinois, the jail had the look of a historical site. Cells lined a long, antiquated marble hallway leading to a large circular steel table where inmates socialized, and in the corner, above the table and just out of reach, was a television. "We had to climb on the table to change the channel," Becca later remembered. Each 6 x 9 foot cell had a commode and a steel sink that gripped the floor, and two metal beds attached to a stout-looking white-brick wall. Sometimes, when the jail was overcrowded, four inmates shared a cell – two in the beds and two on the floor. It was not like the new jail built a few years later, a $15,000,000 futuristic-looking brick and concrete structure on the outskirts of Ottawa. The old jail symbolized Becca's state of mind, when each day was darker than the one before.

Most of the inmates in the old county jail were drug addicts, shoplifters, forgers, or had been arrested for driving under the influence. "Petty stuff," Becca later said. "A lot of them were middle class kids caught for bringing marijuana across state lines to Chicago on Interstate 80." At times, Becca watched television with the other inmates or played a game of cards. But most inmates, while afraid to say so, did not want to be near a "child killer." They kept their distance, not because of what she did, but for what she might do.

On occasion, Becca was able to compartmentalize her emotions, to tuck the unthinkable ones in a deeper unconscious part of her brain, and to enjoy a lighter moment. "There was Tomasena," Becca said, "who was one of my friends at the county jail." Tomasena, while involved with an abusive man, turned to smoking crack, hoping for the high that it surely gave. She had strolled into a gas station in Streator, Illinois one day, all strung out, demanding money from the steel safe. Without a mask or anything to cover her face, she was easily identified and put away. Nine years later, she is about to complete a stint in an Illinois prison for aggravated robbery.

And Karen. "She tried to stop me from carving on my wrists," Becca said. "She lived in Arizona and was stopped on Highway 80 for hauling 140 pounds of marijuana. We had some very deep and sad talks, and felt safe with each other. Sometimes we watched television for hours." There was Thursday night wrestling and a television show they sometimes watched, one that Karen and Becca liked to sing along with, accompanied by the predictable boos from other inmates. But the darker moments prevailed, when Becca sat in the seclusion of her cell crying, sleeping, and rocking back and forth as she fought the numbness that medications mixed with a troubled mind can inflict.

Each day was the same. After a 6:00 a.m. breakfast, Becca returned to her bed until 8:00, when the morning meds were handed out. Next, she took a shower and washed her clothes, followed by lunch at 11:30. Then she wrote letters and took more meds at 2:00 p.m., followed by a 4:00 mail call. Dinner was at 5:00 p.m., more meds at 7:00, and lock-down at 11:00. The mere passing of time pulled Becca from one day to the next.

Chad came once and told her that he would not return. "I got one letter from Chad. He said that he hated me and couldn't stand me, and that I was a baby killer. He said that I wasn't mentally ill, I was just playing games. I wrote him back and said that he was shit for forging my name on social security checks, and that he was worse than me. I even sent him a picture of Dani and told him that he was the reason she was dead." Ruth McAllister, Amanda's grandmother, came one time as well, and Pastor Rickert on several occasions. Janet and Rosaline, and a man named Don, came from the local church to read the Bible and provide spiritual support. "They all said that God still loved me," Becca said.

"I sent lots of drawings to the kids, and asked for their forgiveness. I told them that I was mentally ill. I got letters from my mom. She talked about Dad and the kids, and I sometimes got letters from Aunt Charlotte, Uncle Leroy, Aunt Rose and Aunt Linda. No friends wrote or came to see me. Before Dani died no one thought that I was mentally ill. Now they all do."

It was a lonely place, this cerebral state frequented by the mentally ill; a place unseen by those who looked from a distance. The idea that people now sensed her troubled mind gave Becca an air of satisfaction.

"I saw my attorney maybe six times during the whole ten months," Becca later said. "He didn't like me. Mostly just asked questions and told me how things were going and told me what the psychiatrists had said. He didn't plan any strategy with me. I was just a zombie to him, a life who didn't deserve to breathe the same air that he did." The nature of the crime, and the loneliness and in a windowless cell, led to deep bouts of depression. A ten month incarceration was a test for anyone, particularly someone who was mentally ill.

The defense counselor, on more than one occasion, questioned whether Becca could participate in her defense. As with most states, the judge, prosecutor, or defense counselor could request an evaluation of a defendant's competency. A forensic examiner, usually a psychiatrist or psychologist, would conduct an examination and present his/her findings to the court, followed by a judge's ruling on whether the defendant was competent to stand trial. If found incompetent to stand trial, such defendants would be remanded to a state psychiatric facility, usually for no longer than one year, until they would be deemed competent to stand trial. The Missouri Institute of Mental Health reports that 70% of defendants in psychiatric facilities are judged competent to stand trial within three months, 20% between three and twelve months, and 2% are released after twelve months. If defendants continually fail to reach a competency level, they are released or committed to a state mental hospital if they are considered a threat to themselves or others.

***

His name was Milton Dusky, a thirty-three year old man who assisted two teenagers in raping a sixteen year-old girl. It was in the 1950s, when Dwight Eisenhower was president and the hottest car was a '57 Chevy. It was a time, like anytime, when the brutal rape of one so young heated community outcries to a rapid boil. In Dusky's defense, a psychiatrist testified at the hearing that Dusky suffered from a "schizophrenic reaction" marked by visual hallucinations, and did not understand the gravity of his offense. Despite his mental illness, Dusky was found "competent to stand trial," and was convicted and sentenced to forty-five years in prison. Dusky's case was appealed to the United States Supreme Court, where the 1960 Court ruled that "competent to stand trial" meant that the "defendant has sufficient present ability to consult with his lawyer with a reasonable degree of rational and factual understanding of the proceedings against him." Dusky was later re-tried and sentenced to twenty years in prison.

Some four-and-a-half decades later, the Dusky vs. United States Supreme Court decision continues to be the "competent to stand trial" standard: the defendant must have a factual understanding of the proceedings – not just the charges – and a functional ability to assist one's attorney in one's own defense. The American Bar Association's Criminal Justice Mental Health Standards noted that "the issue of present mental incompetence, quantitatively speaking, is the single most import issue in the criminal mental health field." The ramifications of error are without boundaries. An evaluator's failure to identify an existing impairment could compromise the fairness; an erroneous finding of incompetence could lead to a suspension of the criminal proceedings and to a period of mandatory confinement and treatment in a mental hospital.

Five to eight percent of all defendants in criminal cases are referred for competency to stand trial evaluations(CST), with only sixteen percent of those defendants judged incompetent(IST). Some ninety percent of criminal cases are resolved by guilty pleas and never go to trial, leaving us without a firm basis for establishing a clinical assessment of "competent to stand trial." While psychologists and psychiatrists generally agree on a defendant's overall mental health, achieving a consensus on anyone's competency is more difficult. According to a study by the Missouri Institute of Mental Health, one research project found 98% percent in agreement over CST findings, while another study showed levels of 59.5%, slightly better than chance. Whatever the numbers, the trend seems to indicate that defendants charged with horrendous crimes are more likely to be found competent, leaving me to wonder whether the nature of the crime and the accompanying political pressures unduly influence the forces that drive the judicial process.

Three general approaches are used for determining an evaluation. One is the more traditional psychiatrist or psychologist's interview, another is the forensic psychologist's approach, where the defendant is tested for adjudicative competence, and the third and preferable method is a combination of the two. Sole reliance on test results, specialized or traditional, is never recommended and can be as self-defeating as reliance on a free-form interview with no structure. The Dusky standard requires a determination of one's ability to understand and participate in one's own defense, not in an evaluation of one's mental health. A defendant can suffer from a severe mental illness and still have the ability to understand and participate in their defense. Psychological and behavioral observations do not, by themselves, address the specificity of the *Dusky* criteria. A more structured assessment is needed, something black and white and more easily understood, like the answers in a written test.

Society has a fervor for tests. From early childhood, to adolescence, and throughout adulthood, our history is marked by a series of tests. We have tests for cancer and all sorts of diseases; tests to measure intelligence; tests for citizenship, driver's license, real estate, and insurance tests. We marvel at the near-perfect accuracy of the DNA test, and long for the day when a few electrodes attached to the side of the head will reveal the difference between the truth and a lie. (The American Polygraph Association claims an accuracy rate of 98 percent for a polygraph. Critics boast a more modest range of 70 to 80 percent.)

Many states mandate that the Dusky standard be followed when administering a competence evaluation. To assist in the process, several testing instruments, each with slight differences in design and purpose, have evolved. Some 60,000 Competency to Stand Trial (CST) tests are administered each year at an average cost of several hundred dollars each. Testing is big business.

***

On February 4, 1999, the court found Becca competent to stand trial, followed by a May 20th affidavit written by her attending physician, Joseph Chuprevich, stating that Becca was unfit to stand trial and could not participate in her defense. At the time, Becca's mental state had declined, and the combination of eight different medications had pushed her into a mental fog. She was now on Tegretol, an anti-convulsant; Klonopin, used to control panic attacks; Trazodone, an anti-depressant; Synthroid, for a thyroid condition; Cogentin, prescribed for tremors; Zyprexa, for the mood swings of bipolar disorder; and Serzone, another anti-depressant. The Court ruled that Becca be retested by Robert Chapman, and that she undergo an evaluation by Anthony Caterine, a psychiatrist requested by the prosecutor.

Over the past five years, Becca had been diagnosed with a host of disorders: bipolar, borderline personality, adult attention deficit, obsessive compulsive, and post-traumatic stress disorder. She was taking seven different psychoactive drugs and one prescription for a thyroid condition, and was in jail for the murder of her five-year-old stepdaughter. Seven months after her arrest, she sat in an unmarked police car, as the officer drove the thirty-minute trip from the county jail to Anthony Caterine's office in Peroria, Illinois. Perhaps the view from her window was quiet and orderly, people moving here and there, doing their daily chores; similar to a child-like moment, when you view the ant hill from a distance. But reality was a psychiatrist's evaluation that would help determine whether Becca's trial would proceed as planned, or weather she would be held at a mental health facility until her competency improved.

Caterine administered the MacArthur Competence Assessment Tool (MacCAT–CA), a test used to evaluate Becca's ability to participate in a criminal proceeding, and the Rey 15 memory test, an instrument used to measure malingering in memory. In addition, Caternine studied Becca's history of mental illness, and her contact with people immediately before and after she allegedly committed the crime. Competency required that Becca have a host of abilities: the capacity to understand information and alternative options, to make informed decisions, and to understand the nature of her criminal charges. It was not enough to be tested on one capacity of adjudicative competence. A defendant with a mental disorder might not have an impairment of the assessed capacity, even though other needed abilities were impaired.

The MacCAT-CA comprises a twenty-two item interview for the pretrial evaluation of adjudicative competence, and can be used with both felony and misdemeanor defendants in inpatient, outpatient forensic, and correctional settings, and can also be used to track progress towards the restoration of competency. This instrument implements a vignette format, objectively scored questions to standardize the testing process, and three competency-related abilities: Understanding, one's capacity to understand the legal system and the adjudication process; reasoning, meaning an ability to discern the difference between relevant and less relevant information and to make reasoned decisions during the trail proceedings; and appreciation, defined as the foresight to recognize the meaning and significance of one's legal circumstances. The vignette, a hypothetical offense involving an aggravated assault at a pool hall, is read by the examiner. The defendant, in turn, is asked a series of sixteen questions dealing with the brief hypothetical. The remaining six questions are used to have defendants make comparative judgment about their own cases and to explain their reasoning.

"This is the best tool now available to help a judge or a jury decide if a defendant is mentally capable of participating in the proceedings against him or her," said Tulsa University psychology professor Robert Nicholson, author of Psychology and Law: The State of the Discipline. In 1999, Nicholson and several colleagues at the University of South Florida completed a two year evaluation, funded by the National Institute of Mental Health, to determine the reliability and validity of the MacCAT-CA. Nicholson and his colleagues concluded that the instrument provided the courts with an accurate description of the defendant's legally relevant abilities, leaving the ultimate decision in the hands of the judge.

A November 2006 article in The Journal of the American Academy of Psychiatry and the Law, by Debra A. Pinals, Chad E. Tillbrook, and Denise L. Mumley, came to a similar conclusion, that the MacCAT-CA, when compared with earlier instruments, "does a more thorough job of sampling relevant competence-related abilities..." The instrument allows for an "objective, standardized assessment of factual understanding, appreciation, and reasoning related to the legal process." But the authors pointed out limitations as well. The structured administration limited the flexibility offered the examiners to probe into areas where the defendant showed deficits; the tool did not explore the defendant's ability to consult with counsel and the vignette may not reveal the defendant's views of his/her own case, both critical to the *Dusky* standard.

In the Pinals, Tillbrook, and Mumley study, fatigue sometimes made the defendants appear to lack reasoning and appreciation, and the instrument lacked the capacity to assess specifically for malingering. "I don't know" responses were returned by certain defendants who genuinely did not know the information or were thought to be malingering or showing poor effort; defendants, particularly those with high degrees of irritability or impatience, sometimes expressed frustration and annoyance at the hypothetical scenario because it was not relevant to their particular legal situation.

Except for a highly scientific test, like DNA, where human error is minuscule and data is pure, the MacCAT-CA is subject to the bias and prejudices of the evaluator, who must decide whether and how to incorporate the test results into a written report; clinical judgments sometimes trump test results. The MacCAT-CA was viewed as one in many such testing instruments that could be used as a supplement in competence evaluations.

Caterine said that Becca scored no impairment on the appreciation section, mild impairment on the understanding portion, and significant impairment on the reasoning section. He used the Rey 15 memory instrument to test for memory malingering and to determine if Becca was exaggerating or fabricating her mental symptoms. According to Caterine, the Rey test, developed in 1964, and considered suspect by many authorities, indicated that Becca was feigning a lack of understanding, and that the results of the MacCAP-CA test were due to her lack of effort, not her mental illness. While Caterine believed that Becca was mentally ill and suffered from a severe personality disorder, he said that she was competent to stand trial.

On December of 1998, Chapman had interviewed Becca, studied her history of mental illness, and administered the Minnesota Multiphasic Personality Inventory-2 test. At the time, he, too, found her to be mentally ill but competent to stand trial. But now, in June of 1999, while Chapman maintained his original claim that Becca suffered from numerous disorders – bipolar, borderline personality, adult attention deficit, obsessive compulsions, and post-traumatic stress – he believed that her competency had deteriorated, leaving her unable to participate in her defense. He further believed that Becca's competency could be acceptable within one year, if treated in a mental hospital.

If Becca was found incompetent to stand trial, she would have been remanded to a state mental health facility, and periodically tested to determine if her competency had improved to an acceptable level. A finding of incompetence could not have been raised in her trial, and could not be used in her defense. It would have been a short-term postponement of the inevitable: Becca would stand trial. For the prosecutor, it would have slowed the judicial process, inviting community outcries and calls for swift justice. From the defense's perspective, a delay might have removed, or at least limited, the possibility of a miscarriage of justice; better to err on the side of caution. But the jury rejected the Chuprevich and Chapman arguments, and, instead, chose Caterine's belief that Becca was competent to stand trial. The long wait was almost over. Two months later, on August 1999, Becca stood trial for the murder of Dani Bivens.

Crazy or Not

It was a medium-sized brown envelope with an exhibit number etched in the right hand corner. Tucked inside were a series of 5x7 inch photographs of Dani, taken before and after her death. I remembered another time when I had seen such photos of my friend who was stabbed to death with a butcher knife. She had been killed by a large man swallowed by a drug-induced rage, inflicting multiple stab wounds from her navel to her neck. That image has never left my mind, not even for a second. The first photo of Dani showed her lying on a hospital bed with her eyes closed and the tube from a life-support system taped securely to her mouth. Her blond hair was slicked back towards the top of her head, as if her face had been wiped with a cool wet cloth. A black-and-blue bruise covered her right eye and a portion beyond. It was obvious that she had been hit by a very large fist. Despite the tube and tape and battered face, I was struck by her child-like beauty.

Three photos were taken after Dani's death: Two were of her body resting on what appeared to be a doctor's table covered with a white sheet. Bruised imprints of someone's left and right thumbs were embedded into her flesh, reaching from the armpits up to the shoulders. Someone had picked her up, and with a firm grip, shook and squeezed the life out of her. A third photo, the most unusual of all, was of a blood-soaked brain, resting inside a human skull.

I tried to comprehend what I had seen, but I froze. It was one of those uncommon moments when a queasiness rushed through my body, causing me to hesitate while I wondered if I would be sick. My mind struggled to process what I saw, much like a computer labors when it downloads an unusually large file. How could something so awful happen to someone so pure? Does this change my feelings towards Becca? But my compassion for Becca never wavered. The violence committed upon Dani was not perpetuated by Becca, the woman I had gotten to know. Perhaps it was the shell of a person who looked like Becca, someone filled with a rage that powered her through a senseless act, someone who lacked, for a few moments, any semblance of sanity. Perhaps it was the octopus-like creature, the one that I had imagined. Perhaps.

I could only imagine the effect that Dani's photographs had on the jury. Some might have pushed for a quick justice, pleaded for retribution, or felt an unfamiliar blend of sadness and rage. The prosecution wanted the jurors to see, and possibly touch the photos, while the defense dreaded the prejudicial influence of such an experience. How often have we heard "a picture is worth a thousand words?" The visual potency of a series of disturbing photos has a more profound influence on the brain than a series of spoken words. No amount of talking could dull the image of Dani's battered face. Trips to the judge's bench, where the prosecutor and defense attorney argued their positions in whispered tones, gave them hope that the judge might rule their way. After screening the photos, weighing their relevance, the judge came to the conclusion that the photos were admissible evidence, and would be seen by the jurors. While understandable, this was a heavy blow to the defense.

The defense attorney, Becca's family and friends, never questioned whether Becca killed her five-year-old step-daughter. A signed confession written in her own handwriting, even though she doesn't remember doing it, provided the evidence needed to nail Becca with the crime. The ensuing trial dealt with Becca's state of mind before, after, and at the time of the murder. It was all about her mental illness. Was she crazy or not?

***

The McNaughtan rules (1843) A person may be insane if "at the time of the committing of the act, the party accused was laboring under such a defect of reason, arising from a disease of the mind, as not to know the nature and quality of the act he was doing, or, if he did know it, that he did not know what he was doing was wrong."

M'Naghten's Case, 10 Clark & Fin.

210, 8 Eng. Rep. At 722

It was Friday, January 20, 1843, when Daniel McNaughtan, a thirty-three-year-old stout Scotsman of average height, walked from Charing Cross to Downing Street. A typical afternoon in London – men, women, a few horse-drawn carriages, and the occasional stray dog moved along Downing, a street lined with two, three, and sometimes four-story brick structures – was about to change. In a sliver of a second, McNaughtan's actions changed how the United States' judicial system would view the insanity plea for the next one-hundred-and-fifty years.

McNaughtan approached Edmund Drummond from behind, so the story goes, and pushed the muzzle of his pistol into Drummond's back and fired. Drummond fell to the ground. While McNaughtan returned the recently-fired pistol to his breast pocket and pulled out a loaded one, a nearby policeman lunged at NcNaughtan and wrestled him to the ground, causing the second pistol to fire erratically into the air. McNaughtan was shackled and taken to jail. Drummond was treated by a physician who removed the steel ball that had lodged under the lowest left rib next to the skin's surface. The next morning Drummond experienced breathing difficulties, and upon further examination, it was determined that the rib had been shattered, and the wound had become inflamed. In an effort to treat the inflammation, the physicians extracted a quantity of blood from Drummond's temporal artery, and a large number of leeches were applied to his back. On Monday, two days later, his condition worsened and he was bled again. On Wednesday, Drummond died.

Friday, the day of the shooting, when McNaughtan was taken to the police station, he was asked about the identity of the person he had shot. "It is Sir Robert Peel is it not?" he replied. In his haste to right his perception of social injustice, McNaughtan had mistakenly shot Edmund Drummond, private secretary to Prime Minister Sir Robert Peel, his intended target. McNaughtan's statement reflected the depth of his paranoia.

> *The Tories in my native city have compelled me to do this. They follow, persecute me wherever I go, and have entirely destroyed my peace of mind. They followed me to France, into Scotland, and all over England. In fact, they follow me wherever I go. I cannot sleep nor get no rest from them in consequence of the course they pursue towards me. I believe they have driven me into a consumption. I am sure I shall never be the man I was. I used to have good health and strength but I have not now. They have accused me of crimes of which I am not guilty, they do everything in their power to harass and persecute me; in fact, they wish to murder me. It can be proved by evidence. That's all I have to say.*

Cherry Blossoms & Barren Plains

Richard Moran, author of <u>Knowing Right from Wrong: The Insanity Defense of Daniel McNaughtan</u>, believed that McNaughtan's attempted assassination of Tory prime minister, Sir Robert Peel, was a reflection of the political and economic climate of early Victorian England. "Rapid industrialization, class antagonism, economic exploitation, and social deprivation – not personal pathology – played the significant role."

<u>The London Times</u> worried over the stigma that the murder might leave on the national character; <u>The Illustrated London News</u> stressed "a need for retributive justice;" and <u>The Morning Herald</u> argued that even if McNaughtan was insane, he was not excused from being held responsible for his actions. <u>The Manchester Courier</u> said that the assassination was the result of the political violence of the day, and that other assassination threats had been made by activist groups; <u>The Standard</u> argued that whether McNaughtan was insane or not, it was a politically motivated murder; and <u>The Glasgow Herald</u>, a Scottish newspaper wanting to deflect ill-will towards their fellow countrymen, called McNaughtan an incurable lunatic and not responsible for his actions.

On Friday, March 3, 1843, Daniel McNaughtan stood trial for the murder of Edmund Drummond. Sir William Follett, solicitor general, represented the prosecution, while Alexander Cockburn led the defense team. Chief Justice Tindal, assisted by Justice Williams and Justice Coleridge, presided at the trial.

Through a series of witnesses, Follett established a narrative that McNaughtan had killed Drummond. And the fact that Sir Robert Peel was the intended target did not lessen the crime. The murder was the result of an "ill-regulated mind," so he said, "worked upon by morbid political feelings." Anticipating an insanity plea, Follett told the jury that they needed to consider the defendant's state of mind at the time he committed the crime. "If you believe that when McNaughtan fired the pistol, he was incapable of distinguishing between right and wrong..., that he did not know he was violating the law both of God and man: then undoubtedly, he is entitled to your acquittal." Follett went on to explain that if the defendant committed the act under partial insanity, that his disease was confined to politics, then according to the "principles of the English law" the jury must bring a verdict of guilty.

Cockburn, attorney for the defense, asked the jury to show proper respect for the medical experts, and to consider the fact that past judicial treatment of the mentally ill was formed without the benefit of modern medical knowledge. "Madness is a disease of the body operating upon the mind...and a precise and accurate knowledge of this disease can only be acquired by those who have spent a lifetime in its study." Cockburn went on to explain how the mind is divided into two separate parts: one houses the intellect – the perceptions, judgment, and reasoning; the other holds the moral faculties – the sentiments, affections, propensities, and passions. While one section might be subject to disease, the other could be healthy. One diseased section might make a man "the victim of the most fearful delusions." The fact that the defendant was able to formulate and carry out his plan did not mean that he was sane. It was his moral side, not his intellect, that was without reason.

Cockrun called both lay and professional witnesses. The lay witnesses contended that McNaughtan suffered from delusions of persecution almost two years prior to the assassination of Drummond. The professional witnesses, led by Dr. Edward Thomas Monro, examined McNaughtan four weeks after his arrest. Monro maintained that the defendant's moral faculties were impaired by his "extraordinary delusion." Monro testified that for McNaughtan, everything was done by signs: that encountering a man on the street carrying an armful of straw meant that he was destined to "lie upon straw in an asylum." The defendant received a "scowling look" from the victim as he passed on the street, another sign that aroused feelings of past persecution. Shooting Drummond gave McNaughtan much needed relief.

After several additional medical witnesses supported Monro's diagnosis, Justice Tindal asked Follet if he had any expert witnesses to contradict the defense. When Follet answered no, Tindal said; "We feel the evidence, especially that of the last two medical gentlemen...who are strangers to both sides and only observers of the case, to be very strong, and sufficient to induce my learned brother and myself to stop the case."

Justice Tindal told the jury that all of the medical evidence seemed to support one side, and that he questioned whether it was necessary to go through the other evidence. "If you think the prisoner capable of distinguishing between right and wrong, then he was a responsible agent and liable to all the penalties the law imposes...If not so,...then you will probably not take upon yourselves to find the prisoner guilty. If you think you ought to hear the evidence more fully...I will state it to you, and leave the case in your hands."

The jury foreman answered, "We require no more, my Lord."

"If you find the prisoner not guilty, on the ground of insanity...proper care will be taken of him," Justice Tindal said.

The jury did not retire to its chambers. They huddled in a group, so the story goes, and exchanged brief whispers that McNaughtan did not know what he was doing. After retiring to their chairs, the foreman stood and addressed Justice Tindal. "We find the prisoner not guilty, on grounds of insanity."

McNaughtan was taken to the criminal lunatic department of Bethlehem Hospital to "await the Crown's pleasure:" the equivalent of a one-day-to-life sentence. An 8 x 10 foot stone cell, containing a trundle bed, straw mattress, chair, and small table, became his home for the next twenty-one years. Except for one incident when McNaughtan refused to eat and had to be force-fed, he was considered a model inmate-patient at Bethlehem. But his photograph taken in 1856 showed a hardened man with a chiseled face and eyes like petrified wood. In 1864, this troubled man was transferred to the new State Criminal Lunatic Asylum at Crowthorne in Berkshire, where he would reside until his death on May 3, 1865.

Immediately following the trial, the public was outraged, and feared an imaginary group of madmen might kill with impunity. They believed that McNaughtan had gotten away with murder. The Times argued that even if McNaughtan was persecuted the way he imagined, he still should have been held accountable. They further believed that "the judge in his treatment of the madman yielded to the decision of the physician, and the physician in his treatment became the judge." The Illustrated London News added that those who passively indulge themselves in the doctrines of socialism and infidelity and thereby willingly undergo a process of mental intoxication cannot claim to be entirely without legal or moral responsibility. The Examiner questioned how the medical experts could be certain about the state of McNaughtan's mind, while The Weekly Chronicle took the position that the defendant was insane, and that it would do little good to punish him.

Queen Victoria felt that justice had been denied. She directed Sir Robert Peel to push the legislature into requiring the judges to follow the law as laid down by the lord chancellor. In response to her concerns, the House of Lords took up the question of criminal responsibility, particularly in the area of insanity. Chancellor Lord Lyndhurst declared that no change in the laws concerning insanity was necessary. He believed that the "only course...the Lords can pursue is to lay down some general and comprehensive rule, and to leave those who administer the laws...to apply that rule." The chancellor then suggested that the judges of the Supreme Court of Judicature be gathered to hear opinions on the law on insanity, with particular attention to the McNaughtan trial. What evolved from those hearings became known as the McNaughtan Rules, which examined three general areas of the insanity law: criminal responsibility of persons laboring under partial delusions; direction to the jury in such cases; and evidence, i.e., medical witnesses present at the trial. Stated briefly: To establish a defense on the grounds of insanity, it must be clearly proven that, at the time of the committing of the act, the party accused was laboring under such a defect of reason, from disease of the mind, as not to know the nature and quality of the act he was doing; or, if he did know it, that he did not know that what he was doing was wrong.

In England, the McNaughtan Rules were the test of criminal responsibility until the Homicide Act of 1957, which introduced the Scottish concept of "diminished responsibility." The Act allowed the jury in first-degree murder cases to find a defendant guilty of the lesser crime of manslaughter, provided the defense could prove by a "balance of probabilities, that the defendant was suffering from such abnormality of mind...as substantially impaired his mental responsibility." For the defense, the choice was clear: A not-guilty due to insanity sentence resulted in an indeterminate, possibly life stay in a mental hospital, while the lesser crime of manslaughter followed a court imposed penalty, most often of shorter duration. After the Homicide Act of 1957, and the repeal of the death penalty in 1965, the McNaughtan Rules were seldom applied in England. In the United States, however, the McNaughtan Rules were followed for over a century.

***

> **The Durham rule (1954)** "An accused is not criminally responsible if his unlawful act was the product of mental disease or defect."
>
> UnitedStates v. Durham 214 F.2d 862.

Becca's mental illness was never questioned, but did she, at the time of the crime, know the difference between right and wrong, as directed by the McNaughtan rules? The prosecution said yes. The defense maintained that Becca, while in a manic state accompanied by psychosis, had lost touch with reality, and was not responsible for her actions. The insanity plea lacked clarity. Clouds of doubt blocked the jury's view, causing some to struggle with the complexities that accompany a simple premise: Anyone who suffers from a mental disease and does not know the wrongfulness of his or her actions, is not guilty by reason of insanity.

While lawyers argue in legal terms – insanity is a legal, not a medical concept – psychiatrist's reason in the scientific language of behavioral and cognitive psychiatry. Psychiatrists often complain about being asked, sometimes months after the act, to determine whether a defendant knew the difference between right and wrong, to determine a moral question rather than an evaluation of the defendant's mental competency. How could the jury be certain that Becca, or any defendant, was insane when they committed a crime? Add the disturbing photos of a brutal crime, and the sadness and anger feeds on confusion like a school of Pirana. The jury, saddled with their personal bias, is left to judgments based on the quality of counsel, the attitude of the trial judge, and the salesmanship of the expert witnesses. Becca's fate was determined by a not-so-exact science.

The insanity plea has been tinkered with and tweaked for more than a century. Perhaps a different word, or an altered phrase, would sharpen the definition of insanity. The first significant change came in 1953, when Monte Durham, a 23 year old man who had been in and out of prison and mental institutions for the past four years, was convicted for housebreaking. Although the defense failed to convince the judge that Durham did not know the difference between right and wrong at the time of the act, Durham's case was appealed on a technicality, and reached the Appellate court. Citing leading psychiatrists and jurists of the day, the appellate judge – determined to right the McNaughtan rules – stated that McNaughton was based on "an entirely obsolete and misleading conception of the nature of insanity."

Justice Leventhall, Circuit Judge for the United States Court of Appeals, expressed concerns that McNaughtan's language on the right/wrong provision for insanity was out-dated, no longer reflecting the community's judgment as to who ought to be held criminally liable. The Durham rule more accurately reflected the "sensibilities of the community as revised and expanded in the light of continued study of abnormal human behavior." But critics complained that Durham lacked specificity, allowing alcoholics, compulsive gamblers, drug addicts, and the like, to successfully use the defense to avoid a variety of crimes.

***

> **The Brawner rule (1972)** A defendant is not responsible for criminal conduct where he, as a result of mental disease or defect, did not possess "substantial capacity either to appreciate the wrongfulness of his conduct or to conform his conduct to the requirements of the law."
>
> United States v. Brawner 471 F.2d 969

It was 1972, so the story goes. After a morning and afternoon of heavy drinking, Archie W. Brawner Jr., went to a party, where he was injured in a fight that broke out in the evening hours. Brawner, beaten and alone, left the party and told some friends that several men jumped him, and that someone was going to pay. Minutes later, he returned to the party, entered the apartment building, moved down the hallway, and shot several times into a metal door. One of the bullets pierced the door and hit Billy Ford, who fell to the floor and died.

At the trial, a friend testified that Brawner "looked like he was out of his mind." Expert witnesses, called by both the defense and prosecution, agreed that Brawner suffered from a disease of "psychiatric" or" neurological" nature. But the experts could not agree on what part the mental disease or defect played in the murder of Billy Ford.

Brawner's case was later heard by the United States Court of Appeals for the District of Columbia Circuit, which argued that the Durham rule was too restrictive, and should give more power to the juries. What became known as the Brawner rule was based in large part on the American Law Institute's (ALI) Model Penal Code, which said that a defendant is not responsible for criminal conduct where he, as a result of mental disease or defect, did not possess "substantial capacity either to appreciate the criminality of his conduct or to conform his conduct to the requirements of the law."

Although subtle in appearance, the changes were significant. The substitution of the word "appreciate" for the word "know," as used in McNaughtan, showed that a sane offender must be emotionally as well as intellectually aware of the significance of his conduct. The use of the word "substantial" was meant to respond to recent case law developments that required showing total impairment for exculpation from criminal responsibility. Brawner broadened the definition of mental impairment used in McNaughtan, including both the cognitive and emotional aspects of mental illness.

***

The Insanity Defense Reform Act of 1984 (U.S.)
A person accused of a crime can be judged not guilty by reason of insanity if "the defendant, as a result of a severe mental disease or defect, was unable to appreciate the nature and quality or the wrongfulness of his acts."

March 31, 1981. Ronald Reagan, 40th President of the United States, finished a speech pushing his economic program and deploring the rising violent crime in the inner cities. Surrounded by secret service agents, metropolitan police, and white house staff, Reagan left the Washington Hilton Hotel and hurried through a light rain toward a limousine parked some twelve feet away. It was 2:25 p.m., so the story goes, when Reagan, looking very presidential with his Reaganistic smile, and a slightly cocked head that was a staple in his movies, waved to a hundred or so well-wishers standing behind a roped-off area. Reporters readied for a story; cameramen wanted that special photo; and a patchwork of people waited for a glimpse of their President. It was a scene that would be replayed countless times on the daily news, and discussed on every talk show across the nation.

It was sudden, like a flock of black birds in startled flight. Gunshots pierced the air, six of them. Bang, bang, and then a pause, followed by four successive shots fired from within the crowd. It appeared as though the President had not been hit. Secret service agents had pushed him into the car. But an eye witness, as reported by Lou Cannon of the <u>Washington Post</u>, said it all; "The President winced. The smile just sort of washed off his face." Three men fell to the ground – Timothy J McCarthy, a secret service agent, Thomas Delahanty, a metropolitan policeman, and James Brady, the likeable press secretary who friends called "the bear." While McCarthy and Delahanty each had flesh wounds, Brady took a bullet to his head. Rain washed puddles of blood down the sidewalk and onto the road. Agents pounced upon a white, blond haired man, later identified as John Hinckley, a twenty-nine year old dressed in a raincoat, blue shirt, and dark trousers, who gripped an automatic handgun while they wrestled him to the ground. Hinckley was then subdued and whisked off to jail. The President's limousine and police cars raced to the George Washington University hospital.

President Reagan's wound was serious: a .22 slug penetrated his chest, ricocheted off a rib, and entered his lung, resting about one inch from his heart. An eighty-minute surgery followed by twelve days in the hospital led to a full recovery. McCarthy and Delahanty recuperated as well. But Brady was not as fortunate. The bullet seemed to explode in his head, causing permanent brain damage.

Numerous eye witnesses and a video recording left no doubt that John Hinckley was the shooter. Initial public speculation centered on whether Hinckley would spend the rest of his life in prison, or if he would be put to death. But as days passed, Hinckley's future became less certain. His mental state began to unfold. In 1976, five years before the shooting, Hinckley became obsessed with the movie <u>Taxi Driver,</u> where a psychotic taxi driver, Travis Bickle (played by Robert DeNiro), contemplates political assassination and then rescues a young prostitute, Iris (played by Jodi Foster), from a pimp. Hinckely took on the mannerisms – the army fatigue jacket, the fascination with guns, and even the taste for peach brandy – of the Bickle character. Hinckley's infatuation with Iris developed into a full-fledged imaginary love for Jodi Foster, so much that he sent her love letters and stalked her on the Yale university campus. It was later revealed that Hinckley had even stalked President Carter and planned to assassinate him to impress Jodi Foster. But each time, he was unable to follow through on his original intent. A love letter sent to Foster just hours before he carried out his assassination attempt of Ronald Reagan showed the depth of Hinckley's mental illness.

> *Dear Jodi,*
> *There is a definite possibility that I will be killed in my attempt to get Reagan. It is for this very reason that I am*

writing you this letter now.

As you well know by now I love you very much. Over the past seven months I've left you dozens of poems, letters and love messages in the faint hope that you could develop an interest in me. Although we talked on the phone a couple of times I never had the nerve to simply approach you and introduce myself. Besides my shyness, I honestly did not wish to bother you with my constant presence. I know the many messages left at your door and in your mailbox were a nuisance, but I felt that it was the most painless way for me to express my love for you.

I feel very good about the fact that you a least know my name and know how I feel about you. And by hanging around your dormitory, I've come to realize that I'm the topic of more than a little conversation, however full of ridicule it may be. At least you know that I'll always love you.

Jodi, I would abandon this idea of getting Reagan in a second if I could only win your heart and live out the rest of my life with you, whether it be in total obscurity or whatever.

I will admit to you that the reason I'm going ahead with this attempt now is because I just cannot wait any longer to impress you. I've got to do something now to make you understand, in no uncertain terms, that I am doing all of this for your sake! By sacrificing my freedom and possibly my life, I hope to change your mind about me. This letter is being written only an hour before I leave for the Hilton Hotel. Jodi, I'm asking you to please look into your heart and at least give me the chance, with this historical deed, to gain your respect and love.

I love you forever,
John Hinckley

The insanity law at the time of the shooting provided that an accused was not criminally responsible for his act if, at the time of the commission of the crime, the defendant, as a result of mental disease or defect, "lacks substantial capacity to appreciate the wrongfulness of his conduct or to conform his conduct to the requirements of the law." Vincent J. Fuller, the lead attorney for the defense, said that their challenge was to show that Hinckley did not "appreciate" the "wrongfulness" of his conduct. The psychiatrists for the prosecution concluded that Hinckley was legally sane – that he appreciated the wrongfulness of his act – at the time of the shooting, while the psychiatrists for the defense testified that Hinckley was psychotic – and legally insane – at the time of the shooting. The lead psychiatrist for the defense said that Hinckley had "an incapacity to have an ordinary emotional arousal, autistic retreat from reality, depression including suicidal features, and an inability to work or establish social bonds." Hinckley was schizophrenic.

John Hinckley was found not guilty by reason of insanity. The public outcry was fast and furious. Less than one month after the trial, congress flexed it's muscle and held hearings on the insanity plea. The emotional shock and anger in the attempted assassination over a popular sitting president, and the not guilty verdict, caused congressional leaders to create laws based more on polls than on common sense. What happened over the next three years were limitations of the insanity plea, requiring the use of the word "severe" mental disease, and replacing "unable to appreciate" with "lacks substantial capacity"; a shifting of the burden of proof from the prosecution to the defense; stricter procedures governing the hospitalization and release of defendants; and limiting psychiatric testimony by enacting a statute stating that "No expert witness testifying with respect to the mental state or condition of a defendant in a criminal case may state an opinion or inference as to whether the defendant did or did not have the mental state or condition constituting an element of the crime charged or a defense thereto. Such ultimate issues are for the trier of fact alone." Three states – Utah, Montana, and Idaho – abolished the insanity defense.

In 1984, Congress passed, and President Ronald Reagan signed, the Comprehensive Crime Control Act. The federal insanity defense now required the defendant to prove, by "clear and convincing evidence," that "at the time of the commission of the acts constituting the offense, the defendant, as a result of a severe mental disease or defect, was unable to appreciate the nature and quality or the wrongfulness of his acts." The insanity defense seems to have made a full circle back to the McNaughtan rules of 1843: the "knowing right from wrong" standard.

Another byproduct of the debate was the "guilty but mentally ill" (GBMI) verdict, which was adopted by twelve states. (By 2000, twenty states used GBMI). While the defendant is considered guilty of the crime, he is judged to be mentally ill, and therefore entitled to mental health treatment while institutionalized. If the defendant recovers, he will spend the remainder of his sentence in prison. The National Alliance on Mental Illness (NAMI), opposes the GBMI statue because the statue punishes rather than treats the person with a serious mental illness who committed a crime as a consequence of their illness. For Becca, the GBMI verdict led to six months in the mental health unit at the Dwight Correctional Center, and then a transfer into the general population to live out the remainder of her sentence. The psychological treatment was sparse. "They don't care about us," Becca said. "You have to beg for help."

It can be argued that the GBMI is a compromise, possibly a copout, no longer requiring the jury to make the difficult choice between guilty or not guilty by reason of insanity. Ralph Slovenko, Professor of Law and Psychiatry at the Wayne State University Law School in Detroit, said that "guilty but mentally ill is a sham. It is nothing more nor less than another guilty verdict." According to Slovenko, the jury has the misconception that the defendant will receive special treatment for his illness. Instead, the guilty, and the guilty but mentally ill, are sent to the same prison. Meaningful treatment is not the reality.

At the trial, there was never any doubt that Becca had killed Dani. Still, I would have felt more convinced of Becca's guilt if the interview that led to her confession had been audio or video recorded. Although the interrogation room had the capability for such recordings, none were taken. I would have felt more assured if the fingerprints from the bruises on Dani's body had been shown to match Becca's, or if there were any forensic evidence linking Becca to the crime. (Maybe I just have a more questioning nature). We were left with the confession of a woman, who everyone, defense and prosecution included, believed to be mentally ill.

Joseph Chuprevich, the defendant's attending physician, and Robert Chapman, who had examined Becca on two occasions, one in February of 1999 and again in June of 1999, said that Becca suffered from bipolar disorder, a disorder that greatly weakens an individual's ability to control behavior. Both agreed that Becca did not know what she was doing at the time of the crime.

Anthony Caterine disagreed. Based on a single interview of Becca, Caterine concluded that Becca appreciated the criminality of her conduct, that she suffered from a borderline personality disorder, causing her to become enraged by the victim's rejection of her as a mother. Caterine also believed that Becca was not bipolar, which was a contradiction to Chuprevich and Caterine, and four doctors who had treated her for bipolar disorder from 1993 to 1996.

Becca told detectives and hospital personnel that Dani's injuries were suffered when she jumped on the bed and fell to the floor. This lie, according to the prosecutor, Daniel Day, was proof that Becca knew what she was doing when she committed the act. And Caterine's testimony that Becca faked the answers on the MacArthur Competency Assessment Tool, reinforced the prosecutor's claims. (Caterine said that Becca's poor performance was not a byproduct of her mental illness). Chapman countered with testimony that Becca's lies about the cause of Dani's injuries did not necessarily mean that she appreciated the criminality of her conduct. Becca was suffering from the manic psychosis phase of bipolar disorder that substantially impaired her capacity to comprehend the criminal nature of her acts.

The judge gave the jury a choice of verdicts. They could choose not guilty, guilty of first degree murder, not guilty by reason of insanity, or guilty but mentally ill. They chose the latter. Becca was to spend the rest of her life in prison for the murder of Dani Bivens.

Less than one percent of defendants in criminal cases plead insanity, and only one-fourth of them are successful. The majority of those acquitted by reason of insanity are schizophrenic or, like Becca, suffer from bipolar disorder. The insanity defense has become the last choice, an act of desperation, giving only a glimmer of hope for the most disturbed, who, while in a confused state of mind, sometimes make an unconscious choice to commit a violent crime. Throughout history, the insanity plea has been nearly as troubling as the crime itself. Until you have been stung by mental illness, or have struggled with a loved one who lives on the dark side, the mystery persists.

Becca's journey can be as mystifying as a trip to the moon. The photos, the words, the creative simulations that bring us close to flying through space or walking over moon dust, seem like make believe. Traveling to an illusionary world, where neurotransmitters pop and crackle like fireworks on the fourth of July, is even more baffling. Only one percent of the population, roughly 2.5 million people, make the trip. They are so unique that we call them by a different name – bipolar. Becca is one of them.

When I asked Becca what she would like her family, friends, and the people of Streator, Illinois to know about her, she said to tell them that at the time of the crime, she didn't know what she was doing, she was out of her mind. "I can understand how some people might try to use mental illness as a way to get out of trouble. But I had medical evidence. I was in and out of mental hospitals and had a history of black outs. It wasn't like I was faking." She went on to tell me that she wished that Dani was with us. "I miss her so very much and I loved her even more. Just take my feelings," she said, "and put them into words. You're good at that. Make them see that I was sick then, but I'm different now. Tell them that mental illness is for real."

Larry L Franklin

Cherry Blossoms & Barren Plains

Part Two

Larry L Franklin

Cherry Blossoms & Barren Plains

Fish Heads in an Open Bag

Each time I drove the five-hour trip to the Dwight Correctional Center, Becca was on my mind. How could I explain Becca's feelings when she barely understood herself? To ask someone who suffers from a severe mental illness how they feel, is like asking a blind person to describe the colors in the rainbow. The same is true for someone who has been subjected to a series of traumatic events. They both have an innate ability to tune-out, or dull their feelings, so their emotions will be spared further damage.

I remember my first visit to a therapist. She brought up an issue, and then asked me that dreaded question; "How do you feel about that?" When first asked, I was shocked. There is no answer, I thought. It must be a trick question. You feel good or bad. Nothing more. I soon discovered that this was a way of probing into my inner feelings that had been fenced off from my conscious mind. In time, the feelings bubbled to the surface, and a new world began to unfold. Could I do the same for Becca?

I was on interstate 57. To my right was the two-lane highway that was used before they opened the new interstate. An old beat-up truck moved down the worn-down highway. What if Becca was in that truck, I thought. I was one of the many people driving their vehicle down the four-lane highway that day. Each highway – the new and the old – was separated by a wide strip of land. Unaware of what was happening in that old pickup truck, the people on interstate 57 listened to the latest hits, conversed with a fellow passenger, or talked on their cell phone. The highways represented separate worlds, with no communication between the two. It reminded me of what Becca once said; "No one knows how I feel. I live in my own little world."

It was then that I decided to try a different approach. I began writing down what I thought that Becca might have felt when she was off her medications. I asked her to read it and tell me if I had properly described her feelings. There were many times when I failed, but others when I hit a home run. Those were the times when she became excited, and lengthy conversations followed. "You have a way with words," she said. "Keep writing and I'll tell you if it's right."

I have listened to Becca for hours upon hours. In every season of each passing year, I have sat across from her in the visit room, looking at her drawn and tired face, listening to her struggle to find ways of expressing her mental and emotional realities. What she says is not always cohesive, or narratively coherent, but over time, I have learned to piece together the fragments of her mental processes, and the images that she sees, in ways that blend with my imagination. If Becca hears "voices" or "racing thoughts," it might now be said that I do, as well. The voices she hears are sometimes commanding and destructive. But the voice I hear – Becca's own, echoing in my mind long after I have left the prison – is that of a fellow human being, a desperately ill and still-grieving woman, trying to make herself understood. I believe that I understand her and can, in one sense, show what Becca might say if she could find the words.

***

My name is Rebecca Bivens. It was the 1980's. I was barely a teenager and the summer days were long and dry. Bacon was frying in a black metal skillet, and the morning was clear. My mother was talking and pouring her first cup of coffee. Her voice was faint and the words made no sense and the sounds became one, like the annoying hum of a fluorescent light. She probably told me that Dad and my brother were going fishing for the day, or that my room was a mess, or that I was just a bad kid.

I might have been thinking about the fish heads I saw at Friday night's fish fry. The severed heads were stuffed into open bags. The bodies were gutted, washed, and rolled in seasoned flour, and cooked in black skillets like my mother used. The heads were alive. The eyes and mouths continued to open and close, and called out for help. Their misery was real and hard, just like mine. My mother's shouting brought me back to her reality. My mind jumped around a lot in those days. Maybe that's when my mind began to slip away.

***

In the nineteenth century, mental illnesses were viewed as brain disorders. Psychiatrists and neurologists agreed that insanity was a disease of the brain or a symptom of such disorder, and that biological events caused mental illnesses, and that immoral or criminal behavior had no connection to brain disorders. The mentally ill could be pigeon-holed more easily into a single group: people with a broken mind.

By the early 1900's, the National Committee for Mental Hygiene and followers of the Austrian neurologist and psychiatrist, Sigmund Freud, led a movement that merged severe mental illnesses under the broader heading of mental health. Freud, "the father of psychoanalysis," believed that all mental disorders were caused by early childhood experiences, especially those that were sexual in nature, and could be placed on a continuum, with minor behavioral problems on one end, gradually progressing to the most serious mental illnesses – schizophrenia and bipolar disorder – on the other. It was called the continuum or spectrum theory. Becca would be on the far end of that long continuum of mental disorders.

Further into the 20th century, the National Committee for Mental Hygiene continued the movement to prevent mental illness. Drawn to social reform and liberal political thought, the movement broadened the concept of mental health to include those afflicted with a general state of unhappiness; the "walking wounded," they were sometimes called. If patients were untreated, advocates believed that general unhappiness and other minor behavioral disorders could mutate into a more serious mental illness, requiring long-term treatment. E. Fuller Torrey, author of <u>Out of the Shadows: Confronting America's Mental Illness Crisis</u>, believes that the continuum or spectrum theory implies that almost everyone is, more or less, mentally ill, that we've all seen a fish head or two. Research funding and treatment resources, says Torrey, have been diverted to a host of nonmedical problems and social issues. He further believes that mental illness deals with brain disorders and pathology, whereas mental health covers behavior and values. Linking mental illness to social reform and liberal causes pushed it into the political arena, as early as the 1940s.

By the middle 1940's, American conservatives believed that the National Committee for Mental Hygiene and other advocates for mental health were proponents of liberal values, most interested in promoting a social movement. Mental health was too broadly defined and susceptible to interpretation by psychiatrists who were seeking to control our social agenda. The John Birch Society, among others, joined the outcry by saying that "Mental health programs are part of a Communist plot to control the people's minds." Others voiced concerns that the new "values" encouraged immorality and sin, and diminished personal responsibility.

According to Torrey, conservative resistance peaked in the mid 1950's when legislation was introduced in Congress to build a psychiatric hospital in Alaska. Without a proper treatment facility, Alaska had been sending psychiatric patients to a private hospital in Portland, Oregon. Some conservative groups claimed that the proposed hospital would be used by liberal psychiatrists to involuntarily hospitalize conservatives, and other political dissidents. Although the proposed legislation passed, the political opposition to the broader view of mental health had been established.

While Richard Nixon, Ronald Reagan, and the Bush presidencies viewed the concept of "mental health" as suspect, democratic presidents John Kennedy, a key promoter of Community Mental Health Centers, Jimmy Carter, a mental health activist, and Bill Clinton, permanently bonded the Democratic Party and mental health professionals. The issue is now so politicized that support for mental health, however meager it might be, comes only when the democrats are in power. Few legislators are willing to spend political capital for a small minority of the population, who have little money and see fish heads in an open bag.

In 1952, the continuum theory evolved into <u>The Diagnostic and Statistical Manual</u> (DSM-I), the first national system for the classification of mental disorders. The manual provided a means of communicating a diagnosis to the patient, sharing information within the medical community, and providing insurance communities with an acceptable finding and treatment plan. DSM-I was 130 pages long, and included 106 categories of mental disorders. Sixteen years later, in 1968, it was expanded to become DSM-II, 134 pages long, listing 190 disorders. DSM-III, published in 1980, nearly 500 hundred pages long with 265 disorders, caused significant controversy when it dropped homosexuality as a mental disorder, giving ammunition to claims that psychiatry promoted liberal values. DSM-IIIR, a revision of III, published in 1987, was 567 pages long with 292 disorders. Finally, DSM-IV, published in 1994 at 886 pages, includes 297 mental disorders. The growing number of categories has led some critics to question the legitimacy of mental illness.

From DSM-I to DSM-IV, from Freud to Prozac, psychiatrists, psychologists, and social workers have battled for a share of the mental health market. Psychologists and social workers take a more Freudian approach through talk therapy, whereas psychiatrists more closely reflect the familiar role of a medical doctor, who dispenses medications. Although a more subdued turf battle continues, most of the mental health community agrees that a combination of treatments – talk therapy and medication – is the best approach for a fast and lasting recovery. But as a society, we are still tormented by the problematic history of mental illness, laced with myths, fears, and the stench of politics. Our ambivalence has petrified a nation's heart into stone, leaving us indifferent to the fates of people as clearly ill as Becca.

***

The voices have no name. They're not these booming commandments from up above or down below. They're more like thoughts, racing thoughts that pound the inside of my head like a jackhammer. Sometimes I write the words on a piece of paper, and then another, and another. Later, when I'm kind of normal, people tell me that the words make no sense. They stare at me like I'm different, and then they turn and walk away. It's so lonely in my world of cherry blossoms and barren plains. I wish that I could take you on a tour of my brain. All of the twists and turns through the cerebral matter must be a bit like running through a maze. Wherever I turn, I'm always lost.

***

In 1972, David Rosenhan, a Professor of Law & Psychology at the Stanford Law School, pushed the psychiatric community back on its heels when he said, "It is clear that we cannot distinguish the sane from the insane in psychiatric hospitals." Rosenhan's comments were made in response to a scientific study, or a sinister scheme as some might call it, to measure the effectiveness of psychiatric diagnosis. I can only wonder if his idea was the product of late-night brainstorming, or if this was something hatched-up on the spot. Rosenhan gathered an assortment of people – a psychology graduate student, three psychologists, a pediatrician, a psychiatrist, a painter, and a housewife – to carry out his plan to take eight healthy associates, plus himself, and gain admission to twelve different psychiatric hospitals in five different states. Each "pseudo patient" would enter the emergency room, claiming to hear voices that uttered the word "thud." Nothing else, just the word "thud." No other psychiatric symptoms would be claimed. Except for the use of an alias and false employment details, all other biographical details would be truthful. If they were admitted to the hospital, they would then act normal, and say that they felt fine and no longer heard the voices.

Days before the experiment, they refrained from brushing their teeth, combing their hair, and taking a bath. Each was instructed on how to take a pill, first a small one and then a big one, and slide it to the back and to the under side of the tongue, and then, when no one was looking, spit it out. Eight days later, each went to his or her designated hospital, probably a little excited, somewhat nervous, and looking like a homeless person on a bad day. All nine were admitted, eight with a diagnosis of schizophrenia, and one with bipolar disorder, and days later discharged with a diagnosis of schizophrenia in remission. The average stay was nineteen days, with the longest being fifty-two, and the shortest seven.

Rosenhan's findings were published in Science magazine, where he criticized the validity of psychiatric diagnosis, and the demoralizing care each received in his or her respective hospital. Anger blew through the psychiatric community. Most of Rosenhan's critics focused on the ridiculous idea of using fake symptoms and expecting to receive an accurate diagnosis. Giving fake symptoms to a medical practitioner could taint the diagnosis for any medical illness, they said. Robert Spitzer, psychiatrist and critic of Rosenthan's study, wrote, "If I were to drink a quart of blood and, concealing what I had done, come to the emergency room of any hospital vomiting blood, the behavior of the staff would be quite predictable. If they labeled and treated me as having a peptic ulcer, I doubt I could argue convincingly that medical science does not know how to diagnose that condition."

Spitzer, while critical of Rosenhan, acknowledged the need for better diagnostic techniques, and was influential in the writing of DSM-III. Now, some three decades later, Rosenhan is merely a footnote in college textbooks, nearly forgotten by the general public. But that was before psychologist and writer Lauren Slater rekindled the sparks of controversy through her book, Opening Skinner's Box: Great Psychological Experiments of the Twentieth Century. In a single chapter, "On Being Sane in Insane Places," just thirty pages long, Slater hammered away at the psychiatric community. Like Rosenhan, she questioned whether psychiatry lacked the stuff to be considered a science. After all, she concluded, it doesn't have the physiological evidence to back up any psychiatric diagnosis. It is a fledgling science at best.

Slater was so convinced of her notions that she decided to conduct a study of her own. (Well, maybe she did. Slater also wrote a book titled Lying.) She goes through much of the same preparation as Rosenthan himself: slime-coated teeth, greasy hair, a somewhat pungent smell, and a new crop of hair sprouting in her armpits and on the skin of her legs. She stood in front of a mirror rehearsing her line, "I'm here because I'm hearing a voice and it's saying thud." As both a psychologist and a former patient herself, Slater was familiar with the hospital environment, and knew that, unlike in Rosenthan's day, she would not be involuntarily admitted. Three decades after Rosenthan, no one is admitted involuntarily unless they have homicidal or suicidal urges. The question then became, would they give her a diagnosis and would they prescribe medications?

The first was a highly reputable hospital with an emergency room set up specifically for psychiatric issues. Looking somewhat demented, Slater told the attending psychiatrist that she was hearing the word "thud." She experienced no other psychological symptoms, just a voice repeating the word "thud." Ten minutes later, the doctor said that Slater was a little depressed and experiencing some psychotic features. He prescribed the antipsychotic, Risperdal. Feeling somewhat vindicated, Slater went to a total of eight emergency rooms, and in nearly all instances, she was diagnosed as being depressed with psychotic features. She received a "pouch of pills," she would later say, some twenty-five antipsychotics and sixty antidepressants in all.

Slater couldn't wait to call Robert Spitzer, long-time critic of Rosenhan, and maybe gloat a little over her findings. And then, according to Slater, a disappointed Spitzer said, "I think doctors just don't like to say, 'I don't know.'"

"That's true," Slater says, "and I also think the zeal to prescribe drives diagnosis in our day, much like the zeal to pathologize drove diagnosis in Rosenthan's day, but either way, it does seem to be more a product of fashion, or fad."

This is where Slater's chapter ends, but the real controversy begins. Two years after the publication of Slater's book, Robert Spitzer and others have volleyed a barrage of criticism at the truthfulness of Slater's "study." "Someone presents in the emergency room only hearing the word 'thud' and moreover denies being depressed – there's no way that someone is going to say that is psychotic depression," Spitzer told Psychiatric News.

Other critics joined the fray. "It would be nice if she could assuage my concerns about her study by providing us with objective evidence that she did it," said psychologist Scott Lilienfeld.

Psychiatrist Mark Zimmerman was less considerate. "I believe the data were fabricated," he said. Slater said that she did not have the names of hospitals, doctors, or any other data to support her "study," or the claim that she received a "pouch of pills."

What followed was the publication of two lengthy articles in The Journal of Nervous and Mental Disease, one by Spitzer and his associates, and a somewhat surprising response by Slater. She claimed that she never did a "study," and it does not exist. "This is a personal, subjectively written, and consistently casual book about great psychological experiments and my own thoughts regarding them," Slater said. And since it is not really a "study," no supporting data exists.

Slater's initial findings convinced critics of the need for a study of their own. Spitzer contacted 431 psychiatrist members of the American Association of Emergency Psychiatry and asked them to respond to a brief questionnaire, presenting a hypothetical case study designed to mimic Slater's. Seventy-three psychiatrists participated in the study, with eighty-three per cent saying that they would not hospitalize the patient but would instead refer the patient to an outpatient clinic. Those who would hold the patient for the legal seventy-two hour period, indicated that it was for the purpose of further evaluation to make a diagnosis. Thirty-four per cent indicated that they would prescribe an antipsychotic. No psychiatrist recommended an antidepressant.

Slater's concerns about over-zealous psychiatrists who medicate and come up with a diagnosis to match the prescription are noted. But using a "study" that is not really a "study" weakens the argument. Spitzer's concerns, and my own, deal with the possibility that a distinguished writer of Slater's reputation, whose books I have read two times or more, could raise doubts among existing patients or those considering the possibility of seeking psychological help.

Research psychologist Charles J. Meliska expressed his concerns over the reliability and validity of psychiatric diagnosis. "In all studies," Meliska said, "classifying participants as either 'normal controls' or 'depressed' is often more difficult than you might imagine, even though we put a great deal of effort into it, using multiple diagnostic tools to arrive at the diagnosis. And with a disorder like depression (or bipolar, in Becca's case), the mood of the patient can vary markedly from day to day. So, the 'target' refuses to remain stationary, across time."

Without question, psychiatry is not an exact science. But is any medicine without its flaws? How often have we gone to a physician and been diagnosed as having a viral infection? Upon further questioning, the doctor admits that he doesn't really know what we have. Although psychiatry lacks the multitude of physiological tests found in other fields of medicine, progress is being made. Magnetic Resonance Imaging (MRI), Positron Emission Tomography (PET), and Single Photon Emission Computed Tomography (SPECT) are being used to measure neurotransmitters and brain structure. Research is conducted through such studies as The Stanley Brain Collection, part of The Stanley Medical Research Institute. Between 1994 and 2005, the Stanley collection gathered over 600 brains for use in determining the causes and treatments for schizophrenia and bipolar disorder (manic depression). Thousands of sections and blocks of brain tissue have been sent to researchers throughout the world, leading to hundreds of research publications that provide legitimacy.

***

How do you know when you begin to lose your mind? I don't think that you can pick a certain day, an exact time, or even an unusual event. Maybe it's a bit like cancer. One day a doctor tells you that the MRI shows a cancerous growth the size of a grapefruit, and if untreated, you will die. The tumor had been growing for some time, somewhere in your body, unseen by the naked eye.

My mental illness was the same and went undetected until the doctors told me in 1993 that I was bipolar, and if untreated, I would lose my mind. Looking back, I believe it began the day when I saw fish heads in an open bag. But as bad as I felt, I've always had my doubters. Some think that I faked it and used mental illness as an excuse for my violent behavior. Others believe that I'm an agent for the devil. But until you've visited the dark side and felt my torment, I'm here to say that mental illness is for real.

***

"I do not believe that any mental illness exists other than demons, and no medication can straighten it out, other than the power of God," said Doyle Davidson, pastor of the Water of Life Church. (Associated Press story, February 16, 2006.) An attorney for Dena Schlosser, a thirty-seven-year-old mother who killed her ten-month-old daughter, faulted Dena's husband and the church's beliefs for discouraging medical treatment. Dena's husband, John Schlosser, had testified at her trial that he did not seek medical treatment for Dena even when she told him that she wanted to give their baby to God.

Religion has sometimes been cited as a reason for demented behavior. Dena Schlosser, with a history of postpartum psychosis and depression, killed her daughter by severing her arms at the shoulders. As a 1972 Elvis Presley gospel recording of He Touched Me played in the background, God commanded Dena to cut off the arms of her baby. Lisa Diaz, diagnosed as having psychotic delusions, drowned her two daughters because she believed that evil spirits were in her house, and were about to kill her children in a slow and painful way. Deanna Laney, who had experienced five psychotic breaks in the preceding three years, stoned her two sons to death because God told her to do it. Andrea Yates, who suffered from postpartum depression, schizophrenia, and psychosis, drowned her five children to protect them from Satan.

Mental illness is not a disease of the mind, earlier religious practitioners said. They claimed that it was caused by the presence of demons or evil spirits that had invaded a body devoid of the Holy Spirit. Such beliefs undercut the reality of mental illness, allowing irrational fears – and perhaps the ironic presence of actual religious psychosis – to replace the logic of science. Today, the main stream religious community is more accepting of mental health practitioners, and open to their modes of treatment, and has begun to embrace the fact that severe mental illness is a biological disorder of the brain. Still, lingering doubts in the religious community, especially among fundamentalist Christian sects, persist.

Most recently, we have heard from famous actors John Travolta and Tom Cruise, who espouse the teachings of Scientology, an applied religious philosophy, the opinion that psychoactive drugs can destroy the human mind. Travolta went so far as to blame the recent school shootings of Columbine and Virginia Tech on the perpetrators' use of psychoactive drugs. L. Ron Hubbard, founder of Scientology, is quoted in Wikipedia as opposing both psychiatry and psychology, claiming both to be barbaric and corrupt professions. Hubbard teaches his followers to think in terms of the human brain as being divided into two sections: the reactive brain and the analytical brain. The reactive brain holds negative memories that lead to irrational behavior and needs only to be "cleared" to experience true mental.

***

Sometimes they look and ask what's wrong. One day it's a guard, days later it might be an inmate or two. Maybe they see it in my eyes, or maybe they've heard the rumors that wind their way through the prison gossip vine. When they ask, I tell them that I'm bipolar. They just shrug their shoulders and act like they know what in the hell it all means. I think inmates view mental illness the same as the people on the outside. Truth be known, they don't care. But they do give me some space. I think that it's because of my size and the fact that they think I'm crazy. A big crazy person can scare anyone.

***

It was a Sunday afternoon, September 3, 2006, when summer days were at their hottest. The grass was dry, leaves held their last bit of moisture before summer moved into fall. In Montgomery County, just northeast of Washington, D.C., Wayne S. Fenton's body grew stiff as he lay on his office floor. Fenton, a prominent psychiatrist specializing in the treatment of schizophrenia and an associate director at the National Institute of Mental Health, had kissed his wife goodbye before leaving to see a young man whose brain was about to implode. Through his compassion, and his feel for the human mind, Fenton calmed the most psychotic and emotionally disturbed. He had done this many times before. "He had a knack for it," some might say. But nineteen-year-old Vitali A. Davydov thought otherwise, and could not be consoled or convinced to take his medications. He chose, instead, to pound Fenton's face with his closed fists until Fenton could speak no more. Davydov's father, who saw his son acting strangely outside the office door, walked inside and found Fenton's body. Knowing what probably happened, he called the police. With little resistance and no apparent remorse, Dasvydov admitted to having beaten Fenton, and leaving him on the office floor.

Davydov's story is not unlike Seung Hui Cho, who killed thirty-two Virginia Tech students during a shooting spree, or Steven Kazmierczak, who killed five Northern Illinois University students and wounded eighteen more, or the hundreds, maybe thousands, of other killings committed by the mentally ill who were not taking their medications. Such tragedies, and the subsequent frenzy of reported stories, give rise to the perception that the mentally ill are violent people, beyond repair, and should be locked away. Such stories cause many to move to the other side of the street when approaching someone who looks up and talks to the air. "He's probably crazy," they must think. "It's best to stay away."

Patients with untreated mental illnesses, those with schizophrenia, severe depression, or bipolar disorder, are two to three times more likely to commit a violent act – to use a weapon in a fight, or the participation with someone other than a partner or spouse, in fights that came to blows. According to the NIMH's Epidemiologic Catchment Area (ECA) study, approximately seven percent of people without a major mental disorder commit a violent act, compared to sixteen percent who are severely mentally ill. Thirty-five percent of people who abuse alcohol or drugs commit a violent act, while substance abuse among the mentally ill increases the rate to forty-three percent. In each case, the patient was not taking medications. Violence among the mentally ill was independently correlated with several risk factors, including substance abuse, a history of having been a victim of violence, homelessness, and poor medical health. How easy to understand how Becca, while off her medications and beaten by a violent man, gave way to episodes of rage.

Another study measured the prevalence of violence in psychiatric patients during their first year after being discharged from a mental hospital. In each case, the patient's medications were closely monitored. The level of violence among discharged patients, and members of the community in which they lived, were the same. If someone like Becca is taking her medications, under a doctor's care, and is in a stable environment, the likelihood of committing a violent act is rare.

***

It's been nearly ten years and some ten-thousand pills later,

Cherry Blossoms & Barren Plains

since I killed Dani. I can barely say it since I still don't remember doing it. I can't tell you how many times I've thought about it. But each time I try, I end up seeing fish heads in an open bag. Now I try not to think about that part. I just think about what a wonderful girl Dani was. I tell Larry, my writer friend, to write more about Dani. I want everyone to know her like I did. I want them to know how she liked to read books, listen to music, and play make-up. I bought her a long blond hair piece. She loved wearing that hair piece.

I haven't gone completely manic since I've been here. I take my meds every day. I can't take a chance on losing control of myself. But the meds are not easy. I never feel right. My hands shake, I get nervous, and I always have some kind of depression. Sometimes I wonder if that's God's way of letting me know that I'm a bad person. But that's not what my psychologist says. I get to see him one time a month. And that's not what Larry or the Pastor say.

The only reason that I agreed to tell my story is so other people can better understand what happened. And my poor kids who have been without a mother for so many years. I want them to know that I'm not a terrible person as some might say. I want them to know about my world of cherry blossoms and barren plains, and how I sometimes see fish heads in an open bag.

Preventable Tragedies

In the beginning of the twenty-first century, some 218,000 men and women with severe psychiatric disorders are incarcerated in an American prison or county jail. Most committed violent crimes – sometimes murder – while propelled by a crazed mind untreated with medications and therapeutic care. E. Fuller Torrey, a research psychiatrist specializing in schizophrenia and manic-depressive illness, calls them preventable tragedies. Torrey, president of The Treatment Advocacy Center, a national nonprofit organization dedicated to the effective and timely treatment of severe mental illnesses, believes that involuntary treatment can sometimes move the insane to a more acceptable level of behavior, possibly removing the gun from the likes of a Seung Hui Cho, the shooter in the killing spree at Virginia Tech, or Steven Kazmierczak, killer of five at Northern Illinois University, or the countless others who never received proper care – medication, talk therapy, a stable environment. From the fallen victim and his/her family and friends, to the perpetrator, who has family and friends as well, the misery festers through infinity.

"We did not know that Becky was sick," said Anne Kasamore, Becca's aunt from West Virginia. "My sister (Becca's mother) kept it from us when they found out in Illinois, I want you to know that. If we would have known she was sick, we would have all been right there for her. But my sister didn't want nobody to know it."

It was Becca's second trial in 2002, when the court decided whether to reduce her life sentence to something more humane. Anne Kasamore, and Becca's other aunts, Rose Gragg and Charlotte Salley, all testified that they were surprised at the extent of the mental illness that drove Becca to take Dani's life. "I will say this," Gragg said, "I did not know that she had a mental condition but I knew something was wrong because of, you know, just the way she was. I knew something was wrong but we did not know she had a mental condition."

"I knew she had some problems," Salley added. "She had some problems in Ohio. But I was not aware that she had any problems in Illinois." All three aunts looked past the emotional swings between mania and the debilitating depression that led to Becca's multiple stays in the Illinois and Ohio state mental hospitals. While her parents lived in West Virginia, and other family members resided in states nearby, Becca's caretakers were violent men who relished her mania, which led to her promiscuity, and ignored her sudden slides into depression. The preventable became the predictable tragedy, leaving a little girl dead, and a woman sentenced to life in prison.

***

In 2001, after three years of incarceration at the Dwight Correctional Center, the Appellate Court of Illinois, third district, entertained an appeal from Rebecca Bivens, which claimed that the finding of fitness was against the manifest weight of the evidence; the jury's determination that she was sane at the time she committed the offense was contrary to the manifest weight of the evidence; and the sentence should be vacated and remanded because the statute under which she was sentenced was unconstitutional.

The Illinois Appellate Court is divided into five judicial districts, with the third district located in Ottawa, Illinois. Any defendant has a right to appeal a decision of the Circuit Court to the Appellate Court, where attorneys present arguments to demonstrate an error the Circuit Court made in applying the law. They do not re-litigate the facts of the original trial. While the Appellate Court affirms the earlier decision if there has been no substantial error committed in the application of the law, the Court may, instead, reverse the Circuit Court's decision, or remand the case for a new trial, which would then be sent back to the Circuit Court.

While appeals are seldom heard, even fewer give the defendant what they desperately want. But hope is what sustains an inmate. When the opportunity comes, and fate flirts with the tease of another chance, the inmate stews in her prison cell, waiting for a majority of three judges to determine her future.

The Appellate Court first addressed the defense's claim that the finding of fitness was against the manifest weight of the evidence. A statement of facts, as determined at Becca's earlier trial, was the basis for analysis. The Circuit Court judge had been responsible for determining the credibility of the psychiatrist's testimony as well as the defendant's fitness to stand trial, and his decision could only be reversed if the Appellate Court determined that a preponderance of evidence suggested otherwise.

"A defendant is considered unfit to stand trial," Appellate Judge James Lanuti said, "if, because of her mental or physical condition, she is unable to understand the nature and purpose of the proceedings against her or to assist in her defense." Although Caterine differed with Chapman and Chuprevich's diagnosis of bipolar disorder, all three psychiatrists agreed that Becca suffered from a mental defect. Still, Chapman and Caterine had testified that a person suffering from Bipolar Disorder could be considered fit to stand trial. Caterine believed that Becca was feigning the level of impairment caused by her mental condition; Chapman disagreed, believing, instead, that Becca was unable to understand the criminal proceedings against her and reasonably participate in her defense. It was within the province of the Circuit Court, Lanuti added, to evaluate the evidence and determine credibility. "We cannot say that their finding that the defendant was fit to stand trial was against the manifest weight of the evidence."

The Appellate Court then addressed the defendant's claim that the jury's determination that she was sane at the time she committed the offense was contrary to the manifest weight of the evidence. A person is not criminally responsible for conduct if, at the time she engaged in such conduct, as a result of mental disease or mental defect, she lacks substantial capacity to appreciate the criminality of her conduct. The burden of proof, that she was insane when she committed the offense, rests with the defendant. In deciding questions of sanity, the trier of fact may accept one expert's opinion over another. A finding of sanity at the time of the offense will not be overturned on appeal unless it is against the manifest weight of the evidence.

The jury had rejected Chapman's conclusion that, as a result of a long-term mental disorder, Becca lacked substantial capacity to appreciate the criminality of her conduct. Instead, they were swayed by Caterine's testimony that Becca did not appear emotionally disturbed in the hours before the incident; that she did not present any signs of a mental defect when she spoke with medical staff and police officers at the hospital; that she misled officials as to the cause of Dani's death; and, finally, to a signed confession when she was confronted with the findings of the autopsy. Based on the totality of the evidence, the Appellate Court did not believe that the jury's determination that the defendant failed to prove her insanity at the time of the offense was against the manifest of the evidence.

The claim that the sentence should be vacated and remanded was revisited as well. Without discussion, the Appellate Court elected to vacate the natural life sentence and remand Becca's case to the trial court to conduct a sentencing trial. It was not everything that Becca had hoped for, that her verdict of guilt would have been overturned. But she was given a new trial to determine what her prison stay might be. Illinois law mandated a sentencing guideline for the murder of a child to be within the range of twenty to sixty years.

***

May 16, 2002. Barely one year after her appeal to the Appellate Court, case number 98-CF-455, State of Illinois vs. Rebecca Bivens, was scheduled, not to determine her guilt or innocence, only what her sentence might be. The case had been sent back to the Circuit Court in Ottawa, with Judge James Lanuti presiding; Joseph Hettel and Matt Kidder representing the state; and Tim Cappellini for the defense.

Becca's narrative was that of a model prisoner, who acknowledged her mistakes, felt remorse for her actions, and was determined to continue the treatment for her mental illness. James Nielsen, psychiatrist at the Dwight Correctional Center's mental health unit, was the first to testify on Becca's behalf. Nielson had treated Becca soon after her arrival at Dwight, and for the next eighteen months. His diagnosis of Bipolar Disorder I and Borderline Personality Disorder was in agreement with some eight psychiatrists who had treated Becca since 1993. (Caternine had testified at the earlier trial that Becca was not Bipolar.) Upon admission to the mental health unit, Becca had exhibited the mania and deep depression of Bipolar Disorder, and the instability of moods and interpersonal relationships of Borderline Personality Disorder. She was being treated with psychotherapy and pharmacology, and, months later, had shown little evidence of acute symptoms.

The Illinois Department of Corrections stipulates that medication compliance for inmates suffering from mental illness is voluntary, and is left to the discretion of each individual. Each night, just hours before they settled down, hundreds of mentally ill inmates lined the corridors of the Dwight Correctional Center, waiting for their little white cup filled with pills that promised a better way. A month or two later, a vile of blood was drawn from their veins, checking to see if any vital organs were being damaged. The fact that Becca took her medications without pressure demonstrated an acceptance of her mental illness, and a reaching out for proper care.

But Nielson could not give Kidder, the prosecutor, a guarantee that Becca would continue to take her medications if she was released from prison. "I cannot look into the future," Nielson said. There was general agreement that the prison environment offered a degree of stability that was conducive to medication compliance. Without the structure, would Becca remain diligent in her mental health care, or would she waiver, leaving a crack in her armor. It doesn't take much, just a crevice will do. Her emotions might erupt into full-blown mania, followed by the darkest depression. Those were the arguments used to keep Becca locked away.

Gene Peterson, a counselor at the Dwight Correctional Center, testified to the progress that Becca had displayed in group sessions, and through individual psychotherapy. The medications had moved Becca to a place where she was receptive to the behavioral modifications that psychotherapy can provide. While Peterson concurred with Nielson's diagnosis and assessment of Becca's progress, he, too, could not guarantee what Becca might do if released from prison.

Raymond Rickert, Becca's most ardent supporter, the one who stood by her even when family members turned away, testified as well. Pastor Rickert said that he had worked with the prison community over the past forty-two years, and had never seen anyone more committed in improving her mental health. Becca recognized the seriousness of her illness, Rickert believed, and accepted responsibility for taking her medications.

The three aunts – Kasamore, Gragg, and Salley – echoed Rickert's testimony that Becca had accepted her illness, and was committed to stay in compliance with her medications. They pledged their support, agreeing to provide a safety net if Becca was released from prison.

While the defense offered six witnesses to represent their position, the state offered none. Instead, Kidder chose to argue what he thought was a justification for Becca being in prison for sixty years. Kidder spoke of the legal terms, aggravation and mitigation, as he built his case. He believed that the level of aggravation – the circumstances attending the commission of the crime – was excessive. Dani's age, the position of trust and authority from a step-mother, the brutality of the crime, and the impact on Dani's family and friends increased the aggravation of the crime, making a bad one worse.

Kidder argued that Becca's mental illness did not serve as a mitigating factor – a circumstance that might lessen the impact of the crime. While the guilty but mentally ill verdict recognized Becca's mental illness, Kidder said that Becca was not insane. He referred to Caterine's testimony at the earlier trial, that Becca did not have a severe mental illness, and that she simply acted out in a fit of rage. It was just a matter of Becca being mad at Dani because she wouldn't call Becca mommy. Kidder believed that Becca knew what she was doing, and that her mental illness was not a mitigating factor in the commission of the crime. The only assurance that Becca would not repeat her past behavior was to keep her locked away.

While Cappellini agreed that the nature of the crime warranted a charge of aggravation, he said that Becca's mental illness qualified as a mitigating circumstance, lowering the level of accountability. A history of mental illness, in and out of mental hospitals from 1993 to 1996, and the opinions of some eight psychiatrists that Becca suffered from Bipolar Disorder and Borderline Personality Disorder, bolstered Cappellin's argument. Nielson and Peterson had testified that Becca was so ill that she had to be admitted to the mental health unit at the Dwight Correctional Center, proving again the severity of her mental illness. Cappellini asked that Becca's sentence be reduced to twenty-five years.

Before rendering his decision, Lanuti asked Becca if she would like to make a statement. Becca stood, holding several crinkled pages in her shaky hands, and read the following:

> *I would like to first thank God for giving me a chance to be back here again. I know what I've done is wrong and though I might not remember what completely happened, I would just like to say I'm sorry to all those people whose lives I have affected.*
>
> *I have spoken to many people such as psychiatrists, psychologists and my pastor who have become some of the most important people in my life trying to remember what led up to this tragic accident. All I can tell you is how I feel and what it takes to cope with this tragedy every day.*
>
> *To Chad and his family I truly apologize for the pain I have caused you and the emptiness that can never be replaced. To my mother, father and my children, my family and my friends, I truly am sorry for the*

disappointment I have caused in your lives. I never meant for it to be this way.

And, most of all, I would like to say to you, Dani, if there was any way I could trade you places, I would. What I have done to you is wrong but I just want you to know that I would never – if I would have been in my right mind this would have never happened.

I now know how important my medication is to me. I also realized how confused my mind gets without it. I have started counseling 101 and also group to talk about my confusions, my nightmares, and my misunderstandings.

Although it's been three years and seven months, until recently I haven't been able to talk about this tragedy that I have caused without crying. Everyday I still think about Dani, how old she would be, how she would look, and how she would be with the other kids. I know I can never bring her back. There's not a night that goes by that I don't beg her for her forgiveness when I lay in my bed at night.

I can't change the past, all I can do is take responsibility for it. That's why, while I've been incarcerated, I have taken schooling, had a job in the hospital, and have given my support to the girls who have came in as scared as I was. I have not missed a day of my medication, even though it is my choice to take it. If I was sick and could not go to counseling, I would always reschedule. All because of what – all because I want to make a better life for my children and I. I cannot replace the years that I have taken from them, therefore, when I get home, the years we have left together I have to make extra special for all of us.

I'm not saying that I don't deserve to be punished, because I do. I want to take responsibility for my wrongdoings as I have the last three-and-a-half years. What I'm asking is that you understand, people can and do change and I feel with my faith in God and Jesus' hands upon me, I am one of those people who have changed.

But Lanuti, having presided over Becca's initial trial, could not shake the memory that grabbed hold of his mind. He recalled the shocking end of a little girl's life that left an entire community shell shocked. The age of the victim, the position of trust, the brutality of the act, and the impact to Dani's family and friends, he argued, increased the level of aggravation. Although Lanuti sided with Caterine's testimony that Becca was not insane, and knew what she was doing during the commission of the crime, her mental illness could not be denied, and was a mitigating factor. A compromise was necessary, leaving Lanuti with no choice but to pick something in the middle of the twenty to sixty year sentence. Becca would serve forty years in the Illinois Department of Corrections.

Now, in 2008, Becca has served ten out of her forty year sentence. There is no probation, or days off for good behavior; she serves each and every day. An appeal, asking for a shorter sentence, has been filed. Becca takes the medications that dull her emotions, and attends a monthly individual therapy session. She seems to have found her spot – the eye of a storm. The outside world spins around her, seasons come and go, children are born and old people die, all as if she were not alive.

Larry L Franklin

From the City Streets, to the County Jail

In 2006 approximately twenty-five million of them, all colors – black, brown, white, and different shades of hue – came all the way from the spacious plains of Montana to the dairy farms of Wisconsin. Large numbers of them were funneled into lines, moving down a winding path of long sweeping curves specifically designed to reduce stress and suffering. Their vision was restricted to the backside of the one in front of them so they couldn't see what was just around the corner.

One at a time, they were knocked unconscious by an electric shock of three-hundred volts and two amps to the back of their heads. They were then hung upside down by one of their legs. The main arteries in the neck were severed with a knife; blood drained and spurted to the floor; skin was removed by down and side pullers; and internal organs were inspected for parasites and disease. To reduce levels of bacteria, carcasses were cleaned by steam, hot water, and sometimes, organic acids, and then chilled to prevent the growth of microorganisms. There are 5,700 of these places in the United States that employ some 527,000 workers. They call them slaughterhouses.

Although they kill only a few, thousands upon thousands of citizens are systematically segregated from society and kept in holding pens, more commonly called prison cells. Some 2.5 million men and women are prisoners in the United States' criminal justice system. More than half of them have mental health problems, some ten percent having been diagnosed with severe mental illnesses – schizophrenia and bipolar disorder. That's approximately 250,000 individuals – similar to the populations of Madison, Wisconsin or Akron, Ohio – who are incarcerated in the nation's jails and prisons, rather than being treated in a mental institution or an assertive community treatment center, where broken minds receive the care and compassion they deserve.

They come from every ethnicity: forty-four percent are African American, forty are white, and fifteen percent are Hispanic, with the balance made up by various other minority groups. Most are bused, and then unloaded in front of a prison wall. A few, then hundreds, and finally thousands, are assigned an identification number, hosed down, deloused, and issued a set of goose-hunting orange colored clothes. Harnessed with a set of chains, they are herded down a hallway of opening and closing metal doors, leading to a place most have never seen before. Each inmate fades into a distant image, like cattle on a disappearing train.

The criminal justice system has become the largest caretaker of the mentally ill. They have come, in large part, from the closing of state mental hospitals that treated 559,000 clients in 1955, 72,000 in 1994, and only about 38,000 in 2005. Deinstitutionalization was the technical name of the process that systematically moved thousands of people from state mental hospitals to community health centers, where they were promised better treatment than before. But the centers did not anticipate, nor were they prepared for, the long-term demands of the severely mentally ill. Instead, these clients slipped through the cracks, and were left to the care of family and friends, or sought refuge on the city streets. More often than not, they made their way to the county jail.

The political climate in the 1960's, caused by the financial drain from overcrowded state mental hospitals and the concern over the individual rights of the mentally ill, changed mental health laws. Involuntary admission became more difficult. Most states demanded clear evidence that the individuals were a threat to do bodily harm to themselves or to others, or unable to care for themselves. Many individuals, who ignored the advice of psychiatrists and failed to take their medications, walked the city streets, or the dusty roads of their rural communities, or the path that sometimes led to a prison cell.

The influx of people into the criminal justice system was increased, in part, by the nature of the services provided to individuals with mental health problems. Most treatments were symptom specific: limited to alcohol, substance abuse, and illicit drugs. Someone who used drugs to dampen internal torment, was said to have a co-occurring disorder – mental illness accompanied by a dependency on drugs. A center for the treatment of substance abuse, for example, was not equipped to deal with a severe mental illness. The individual was refused treatment, or sometimes fell short of a successful outcome. Drug enforcement, and a commitment by community leaders to rid the streets of loitering, panhandling, trespassing, disturbing the peace, and a host of minor offenses, brought more of the disturbed to the county jails. We were left with a criminal justice system that has become involved in every step, from initial arrest to long-term caretaker for the mentally ill.

Rebecca Bivens, identification number K93737, is one of the

estimated 250,000 inmates afflicted with a severe mental illness. She, like so many others, committed a violent crime that was a preventable tragedy. But that day has come and gone, and now the criminal justice system must deal with a perpetrator who is a victim of a severe mental disorder. The law requires it, says Robert M. Wettstein in <u>Treatment of Offenders With Mental Disorders</u>. The system is mandated by the Eighth Amendment of the United States Constitution to ensure that individuals are free from cruel and unusual punishment. The Supreme Court interprets this to include medical, as well as mental health care to prisoners. While the State can sometimes override an inmate's refusal of treatment if safety is a concern, it cannot impose the use of psychotropic drugs, ECT, and psychosurgery, deemed to be intrusive.

The "seven C's," as described in Wettstein's book, shows the step-by-step process that ultimately determines the mode of treatment that each mentally ill defendant will receive. Crime, catch, charge, court, commitment or corrections, and finally, community, leads us down a logical path of completion, where 95 percent of the mentally ill will eventually make it back to the outside world.

First, the defendant commits the crime and is captured. Charges are filed, followed by a court arraignment, and then the trial begins. If there are concerns that the defendant is mentally ill, the court orders an evaluation of competence to stand trial. A finding of incompetency requires that the defendant be moved to a mental hospital until a satisfactory level of competency is reached. If the defendant raises the insanity defense, the court orders an evaluation of the defendant's criminal responsibility.

Becca followed the process as described. She committed the crime and was captured. Charges were filed, followed by a court arraignment. The court then ordered an evaluation of competence to stand trial, and later ruled that Becca understood the nature of the charges against her, and was able to assist in her defense. After the insanity defense was raised, the court ordered an evaluation of Becca's criminal responsibility. At the completion of the process, her trial began.

If a defendant is considered to be incompetent to stand trial (IST), or is found not guilty by reason of insanity (NGRI), psychiatric services will be provided in a mental hospital operated by the state's mental health system. If defendants are guilty but mentally ill, like Becca, the state provides mental health services most often in a prison psychiatric unit controlled by the judicial system, where they will remain until an acceptable level of mental health is obtained. At that time, inmates are moved into the general population for the duration of their sentences. A guilty verdict sends the defendant to a prison.

Treatment varies depending on whether the individual is part of the civilian population in a mental hospital, a IST or NGRI offender treated in a mental hospital or prison psychiatric unit, or a mentally ill inmate living in the general prison population. With the civilian patient, the focus is on the care and treatment of the disorder. The mental hospital or prison psychiatric unit is concerned with the care, treatment, and custody of the offender, whereas the inmate in the general population is treated with more emphasis on punishment, retribution, deterrence, and rehabilitation.

Becca spent approximately one year in the LaSalle County jail where she received little to no therapeutic care. The occasional visit by a psychiatrist to check blood levels of prescribed medications was the norm. Six months spent in the Dwight psychiatric unit was intended to be more treatment-intensive, utilizing pharmacology, individual and group therapy, with the goal of moving her to the general population where overall costs would be reduced. But the treatment fell short. Not one time did Becca receive individual therapy from a qualified psychologist. She, instead, participated one time per week in group therapy, and met with a psychiatrist every three months for a review of her medications. When asked how she filled each day in the psychiatric unit, Becca said, "I watched a lot of television."

Now, some ten years later, Becca continues to receive the bare-bones treatment offered to mentally ill inmates living in the general population. Every three months she meets with a psychiatrist who evaluates her medication regimen, and runs a blood profile to insure that the prescribed medications are at the optimal levels, not damaging her vital organs. Because of a recent federal grant, Becca, together with other women who have killed a child, participate twice a month in group therapy, plus a monthly individual session with a prison psychologist. When the federal grant ends, Becca's mental health care will be limited to medications, and the occasional meeting with a psychologist if Becca threatens to take her life.

Psychotropic medications are the treatment of first choice. Some twenty-seven percent, roughly 675,000 inmates, pop prescribed pills each day, and wait for the mellowing effect on their brain. Pills make life easier: days pass more gently, nights are quieter, and the bitter memories become more compartmentalized and locked away in that deep-dark cellar of the brain. When the whistle blows for the evening's med line, hordes of prisoners rush to get their fix, knowing full well that without it, the days become longer than before.

For the prison, medications are a godsend. Inmates are more easily managed by the smaller staffs and scaled-down budgets meant to pacify the politicians. But the controls offered through medications can sometimes lead to overly-prescribed dosages to unruly inmates. The agitated become calm; oceans take on the stillness of pond water.

Individual psychotherapy is reserved for the sickest of the sick, and the ones who threaten to end it all. Group psychotherapy, although seldom used, is the most cost effective, and gives the inmates an opportunity to realize that their feelings and experiences are not unique, and that there is hope after all. Group work has been particularly effective in the treatment of substance abuse, an addiction shared by over one-half of the individuals joining the ranks of the prison population.

The harsh environment of prisons can break the strongest. Imagine what it does to the mentally ill. During my time with Becca, she struggled to make it through the four-hour visits without going to the restroom and subjecting herself to another search; she was strip-searched when entering and leaving the visit room, and the restroom as well. I remember the vending machines.. Becca loaded up on everything that her stomach could hold, and marveled at the good-tasting food that bore no semblance to the prison cafeteria fare.

The prison cells, on those summer days when the smell of damp concrete mixed with human odors and day-old sweat, pushed everyone to the edge. Violence bubbled to the surface, only to be dampened by the threat of segregation, or a longer sentence. And then there were the times when inmates received a new cell mate who might be worse than the one before, or get someone they might begin to like, only to have her taken away. The bonding of friends or the closeness where two human beings might touch was forbidden.

Except for the Constitution forbidding the use of cruel and unusual punishment, there are no federal prison standards. It is left to the courts to decide what "cruel and unusual punishment" means.

Cherry Blossoms & Barren Plains

While most prisons have their individual rule book that spells out the regulations and procedures that all inmates must follow, enforcement varies within each institution, as well as the monitoring of any grievances filed by inmates. But there is little effort to avoid the degrading treatment frequently found in prisons today; the emotional trauma, the lack of respect for another human being, and the damage to one's self-esteem has a crippling effect on the inmate's mental health.

Each political cycle calls for harsher penalties, and is as predictable as the change of seasons. Three strikes and you're out; no time off for good behavior; retribution over rehabilitation; and juveniles now tried like adults. In 2005, twenty-three states had no minimum age for criminal prosecution, leaving children to be tried as adults. Two states had a minimum age of ten, three states a minimum of twelve, six states a minimum of thirteen, sixteen states a minimum of fourteen, and one state had a minimum age of fifteen. Some 2500 inmates under the age of eighteen were housed in state adult prisons. Despite the efforts made towards a stronger and more just system, criminals have become worse off rather than better, ready to unleash their violence on others, or simply implode.

Society's well-intentioned philosophers, prison activists, and law-and-order politicians have failed in their efforts to establish a prison system that serves as a deterrent to would-be criminals, while maintaining a rehabilitating experience for the ones who, by choice or circumstance, broke the law. History is full of such mistakes.

In 1829, with the opening of Philadelphia's Eastern State Penitentiary, the nation created what was considered the first state-of-the-art prison, which would serve as a model for the world. All inmates lived in solitary confinement, where they had the opportunity to reflect on their misdeeds, and repent. Prisoners talked only to their warden and the ministers who strolled the prison corridors on Sunday mornings. Black cloths split the center of hallways, blocking the view of other inmates. Although the cells had no showers and the stools were flushed every two weeks, and the cramped cell had a narrow skylight as its only escape from total darkness, the prison was equipped with the ultra modern conveniences of running water and central heat. Compared to earlier times, when males and females, young and old, were thrown into a single room, the Philadelphia experiment was thought to be a more humane system of incarceration. Isolation was intended to provide a monastic environment where hardened criminals would find their soul. But after years of solitary confinement, most lost their minds.

"Isolation breeds violence," Debra Niehoff once said. Those responsible for the Philadelphia experiment were moral philosophers, not biologists, and ignored a fundamental principle of behavioral biology: "Social animals don't thrive in isolation." Biologists believe that isolation wreaks havoc on the neurochemical pathways in the brain, causing aggressive responses to stress. But some two hundred years later, long after the Philadelphia experiment, the criminal justice system continues to repeat the same mistakes: High security prisons have inmates in a twenty-three hour lock down where they eat, exercise, and exist in isolation; inmates who will someday return to the general prison population or be released into the community, are strung tight, ready to unwind at the slightest threat.

I remember when Becca was sent to segregation for a minor altercation with another inmate. She spent three months in total isolation, followed by another three months with a cell mate in twenty-three hour lock down, followed by another month in the maximum security unit, and finally, back to her cell in the minimum security wing. While Becca now has a deep fear of segregation, which some might see as a deterrent to future bad behavior, I would argue that she is more hardened, and less able to make contact with her emotions. Our conversations are less personal and not as free flowing as before.

Prison has a strident lyricism that's never allowed to resolve; song without an ending. New inmates arrive; old ones go; others are shifted, transferred, and regrouped according to some meaningless criteria; unruly ones are sent to segregation and then returned; sometimes you live alone, then with a cell mate, maybe in a dorm. Prison life is in a continuous state of social upheaval that never allows a moment for the soul to heal. As psychiatrist Dorothy Otnow Lewis once said; "Our correctional system reproduces all of the ingredients known to promote violence: isolation, discomfort, pain, exposure to other violent individuals, and general insecurity. In our prisons we have created a laboratory that predictably reproduces and reinforces aggression."

Becca was not hauled to prison in a cattle car or an eighteen-wheeler. It was a police squad car. But she was assigned an identification number, hosed down, deloused, and issued a set of goose-hunting orange colored clothes. Now, some ten years later, she has reached a level of teetering stability, where a regimen of medications and a disciplined environment keeps her in a subdued state of mind. She relies, in part, upon the innate ability of the human brain to protect her. It's as if a psychological cocoon, made of biological magic and spun silk, has encased her emotions, and protects her from further trauma.

Someday, when Becca has served her time, she will face a world without the structure that the prison provides. And like most, she might not enter a passive environment filled with loving family and friends. She might, instead, move into a sometimes ruthless world of stresses and daily temptations; one that she might not survive. E. Zamble and F. J. Porporino in <u>Coping, Behavior, and Adaption in Prison Inmates</u>, conclude that prison life does not provide the coping skills that an inmate, particularly one who is mentally ill, will need. The inmate's psychological behavior remains unchanged, they say, and lacks the maturation that proper treatment can provide.

In Becca's earlier appeal, the prosecutor had argued that Becca could not be trusted to take her medications and continue treatment if she was released from prison. The prosecutor based his argument on the unspoken fact that the system is broken, and does not provide the treatment needed to bring about the desired behavioral modifications. He might as well have said; *If we're not going to help the people, how can we let them out?*

Larry L Franklin

Treatment Works, If You Can Get It

In 1990, when mental hospitals treated some 70,000 people, down from the 559,000 cared for in 1955, and social services felt the cuts of an ongoing recession, the National Alliance on Mental Illness (NAMI) described America's mental health system as "not even minimally acceptable." Sixteen years later the alliance, along with the U.S. Surgeon General, President Bush's New Freedom Commission, and the Institute of Medicine, called it a "system in shambles," an organizationally fragmented image that reminds me of my mother's patchwork quilts.

I remember them well. My mother and a half-dozen or so gray-haired church women circled a wooden frame, sewing different shapes and sizes of little cloth pieces together to form what became the top layer of a quilt. All skillful in their craft, the women scuffled scraps of material into aesthetic-looking quilts that gave me warmth throughout the long winter nights. The mental health system, with all of its fragmentation and bureaucratic structure – a menacing maze for the mentally ill – still waits to be stitched together into that perfect quilt.

Mental health services come from many directions: from the federal, state, city, and county governments, to the educational, social welfare, and the criminal justice system, all supported by medical professions, hospitals, and insurance companies. Providers scurry about, searching for scraps of financial aid, hoping to piece together the funding for another year. But people with troubled minds and broken spirits continue to fill the prison cells; hospital emergency rooms offer a final refuge for the mentally ill; adequate housing continues to decline; and access to treatment is less than before. But when all is said and done, study after study, report after report, patient after patient, show that mental health treatment works, if you can get it.

Someone like Becca, who suffers from a severe mental illness – schizophrenia or bipolar disorder – needs a three-part treatment plan: pharmacology, psychotherapy, and a controlled environment. A psychiatrist develops and monitors a medication regime, where an assortment of pills quell the psychological torment of a troubled mind. The voices begin to stop, the anger subsides, and the racing thoughts slow to a more even flow; the quiet after a storm, when birds can barely sing.

Cherry Blossoms & Barren Plains

A psychologist engages the patient in psychotherapy, commonly called talk-therapy, where a verbal exchange of behavioral issues is shared, and the two begin to bond. Psychotherapy, in its deepest form, is a slow and thoughtful process, requiring months, years, and sometimes a lifetime of treatment. Many psychologists view this as a spiritual journey, where the patient discovers her fragmented soul, and in the exchange, completes a healing process. The patient probes her negative reactions to various stimuli, leading to a better understanding of the origins of such behavior, and how to make the needed adjustments. Each discovery is an awakening – a child-like image, where the child sits on the living room floor, surrounded by books, toys, and a stuffed puppy, and meticulously examines a handful of jelly beans, each with a different shape and color, and a flavor that startles the senses.

Insurance companies and HMO's, more interested in fewer paid sessions than lasting results, have pushed today's psychologists to practice Cognitive Behavioral Therapy (CBT), a more cost-effective psychotherapy. CBT, according to research psychologist Charles Meliska, "is a 'nuts and bolts' approach, in which the therapist tries to identify and replace specific irrational beliefs which generate self-defeating emotional responses with more rational, positive ones." He further explains that CBT has "a more limited goal of dealing with specific self-defeating cognitions and behaviors." While CBT has been used in the treatment of various mental disorders, people who suffer from a severe mental illness, need the more traditional, long-term psychotherapy.

For Becca, as with so many people who are mentally ill, or have been abused, the reaction to certain stimuli is immediate and harsh. Her environment was filled with men who dealt with perceived threats in a violent way – it was easier to hit someone than to talk things out. A fist to her head, a slash from a knife, and sex-on-demand were staples in her life. To navigate such a world, she needed an arsenal of coping skills to disarm what she perceived as threats to her survival. With psychotherapy, and the benefit of time, a new reality evolves, where someone like Becca looks through a different set of lenses, and sees with a new-found clarity. Like pharmacology, psychotherapy can even change the wiring of the brain, causing information to be perceived in a different way. The level of change will depend, in part, upon the severity of the mental illness, the patient's participation, and the skill of the psychologist.

A controlled environment – a peaceful, compassionate world,

filled with the love and support of family and friends – is the final piece of the three-part treatment plan. But what seems so obvious is missing at every turn. Too many Beccas walk the city streets, end up in a prison cell, or live with a family ill-equipped or unwilling to provide the support needed for healing to occur. Each time Becca was released from the hospital, her prognosis was fair to poor. The doctors knew, the hospital staff knew, everyone knew: Becca would step back into a world filled with men who were unaccustomed to a hard-day's work, and strapped with emotional and substance abuse issues of their own; she would have four children to care for, plus babysitting chores and the part-time bartending jobs; and she'd have no support for the continued treatment of her mental illness – no medications, no therapy, and an environment that put her troubled mind through hell. Hardly anyone, mental illness aside, would not have trouble living in such an environment.

Becca's medical records from the Community Hospital of Ottawa and the Ohio State University Hospital tell a similar story: After the initial evaluation, she was given an assortment of pills targeted for the troubled spots of her brain, isolated from family and friends, and treated with individual and group therapy. Days later – a month at most – after a reduction in the symptoms brought on by her mental disorders, she was pushed into the outside world.

How many times have we seen the treatment fall short? An emotional band-aid is applied, and the patient is discharged into a community unprepared to provide the continued care needed for recovery. The Treatment Advocacy Center (TAC), a long-time advocate for the treatment of patients suffering from a severe mental illness, provides a glimpse into the thousands upon thousands of violent crimes that could have been prevented if the perpetrator had received proper mental health care. They list them on their website, as "preventable tragedies." Here are a few.

> On June 7, 2008, forty-year-old David Dunagan shot his twin brother and then killed himself in the McCreary County community of Parkers Lake, Kentucky. State police said the victim, Richard Dunagan, went to his twin brother's house to check on him. While Richard stood at the front door, his brother, David Dunagan, shot him in the head and then turned the gun on himself. David, diagnosed with paranoid schizophrenia, believed that everyone

was out to kill him. He was not taking his medication.

Lexington Herald Leade, 6/8/08

On May 12, 2008, thirty-eight-year-old Brent Douglas Stephens ambushed his ex-wife with a baseball bat. Witnesses told police that Douglas struck the victim, Denise Stephens, as many as twenty times. Denise died at the hospital. Earlier, in 2006, Brent Stephens, diagnosed with bi-polar disorder, slashed his wrists and spent five weeks in a mental hospital. More recently, Brent had rammed Denise's car with his, sent her vulgar text messages, kicked in her back door and stole her phone bill to see who she'd been calling. Less than two weeks before the murder, Brent was convicted of harassment, criminal mischief and criminal trespassing. He received community-service hours and a suspended sentence, and he was ordered to pay his ex-wife more than $1,000 in restitution.

Texas Cable News, 5/13/2008

On February 15, 2008, Cynthia Hernandez shot and killed her fourteen-year-old son, Jeremy Barragan, with his hunting rifle. Cynthia Hernadez, who had attended a barbecue earlier, returned to her home where she shot Jeremy sometime during the evening hours. Cynthia had no recollection of the shooting when she was arrested. Hours later, when she realized what had happened, she broke down and was held in a padded cell and placed on suicide watch. Family members blamed the incident on Cynthia's mental illness – bipolar disorder.

KTAR.com, 2/19/08

Testimony in the first-degree murder trial of Rebecca Bivens concluded late Friday afternoon with a barrage of mental health evidence presented by three psychiatrists, two of whom said she is legally insane and one of whom insisted she is not. Bivens, age thirty-two, of Streator, Illinois, is charged in LaSalle

County Circuit Court with the November 17, 1998 beating death of her five-year-old stepdaughter, Dani Bivens. Rebecca suffered from bipolar disorder and was not taking her medication.
Peoria Journal Star, 7/30/1999

It is not possible to recover from a severe mental illness without pharmacology, psychotherapy, and a controlled environment. When will we see the error of our ways? How many prison cells will we fill before we change our course; how many people will walk the streets; and how many homes will hold the fear that a disturbed family member might slit their throat in the middle of the night? The story of Seung Hui Cho might give us a clue. On April 16, 2007, Seung Hui Cho, a twenty-three-year-old South Korean national, who had permanent residence status in the United States, shot and killed thirty-two people and wounded eleven others before committing suicide on the Virginia Tech campus in Blacksburg, Virginia. Although small in stature, Cho's deranged mind drove him to the crest of a wave of terror that covered a nation that day. The massacre was the deadliest killing spree by a single shooter in my lifetime, and possibly in the history of the United States. For weeks the narrative, together with graphic photographs, filled the cable news. Intermingled within the stories of student lives' cut short, was a glimpse into the mind of a killer who was clearly insane.

When only three, a time when children crave the warmth of a parent's love, Cho was described as wary of human contact; by the eighth grade he had been diagnosed with severe depression and was reluctant to speak; and his middle school and high school years were marked by frequent meetings with mental health counselors. Later, when Cho attended Virginia Tech, his earlier mental health records were withheld from university personnel because of federal privacy laws that prohibit such disclosure. His erratic behavior continued, causing a university professor to seek counseling for Cho. But the professor was told that there was nothing that she could do because Cho was not an "immediate danger." Cho was then investigated for stalking and harassing two female students, and in 2005, he had been declared mentally ill by a Virginia judge and ordered to seek outpatient treatment. Cho never followed through with the ordered treatment.

Images of the bullet-riddled bodies lying on the classroom floors stirred the nation into a near emotional frenzy. *Why and how did this happen?* were the initial questions. The answers were clear, and maybe too simple to hear: Seung Hui Cho was insane, with a reality so shattered that he didn't know, or care, what he was doing; he was not being treated for his mental disorder; and guns were there for the taking. When a calm began to settle on the university campus, additional questions were asked: *Could the killings have been avoided?* Yes. *Who was to blame?* All of us.

Politicians rallied to the public's outcries with speeches, hearings, and promises to protect us from the Seung Hui Chos of the world. Not to be outdone, federal legislators revisited a 2002 bill originally submitted by New York Senator Chuck Schumer and Representative Carolyn McCarthy that required information on individuals prohibited from possessing firearms to be transmitted by State and local government and Federal agencies to the National Instant Criminal Background Check System (NICS). The 2002 bill was originally submitted in response to a church shooting, but never gained the necessary support until the Virginia Tech massacre. H.R. 2640 – the NICS Improvement Amendments Act of 2007 – signed into law on January 8, 2008, authorizes up to $1.3 billion in grant money for states to improve their ability to report individuals who, by law, were not eligible to purchase firearms, including those involuntarily confined to a mental institution. Anyone convicted of misdemeanor domestic violence or adjudicated for mental illness will now be included in the NICS system.

It's difficult to argue against the merits of the federal law – to keep guns out of the hands of the mentally ill. But does it really get to the heart of the problem – to provide treatment for people with a serious mental illness? According to the Treatment Advocacy Center, forty percent of the 4.5 million people who suffer from schizophrenia or bipolar disorder are not being treated for their illness at any given time. That's 1.4 million individuals without basic mental health care. Looking to attack the real problem, Tim Kaine, governor of Virginia, appointed an independent panel to answer two basic questions: What happened to keep Seung Hui Cho from getting the needed mental health treatment, and at what point could the Virginia Tech massacre have been avoided?

The panel inched into a tragedy as fresh as wet paint. When emotions began to build, some panel members probably pounded the table, others might have raised their voices, and some surely wept. In the end, they made ninety recommendations to university officials, mental-health providers, law-enforcement officers, and state and federal policy makers. The panel concluded that "The Virginia standard for involuntary commitment is one of the most restrictive in the nation and is not uniformly applied." The following recommendations dealt with the involuntary admissions of people such as Seung Hui Cho who suffer from a severe mental illness.

Involuntary treatment criteria should be improved to "allow involuntary treatment in a broader range of cases involving severe mental illness." The current standard for the involuntary commitment of someone with a severe mental illness requires the person to be an "imminent danger to self or others" before he or she can be court-ordered to treatment. This makes it nearly impossible to treat someone before they have harmed themselves or someone else, or threatened to do so. The panel further recommended that "reports of prior psychiatric history" be presented at commitment hearings. Current Virginia law instructs magistrates to rely solely on what is happening currently with a person suffering from an untreated severe mental illness. Episodes of violence, psychiatric history, and past treatment are not being considered when a determination is made as to whether someone should be involuntarily committed.

There was never any question of whether people who suffer from a severe mental illness need to be treated, or whether the Virginia legislators needed to improve current laws dealing with involuntary commitment. How to make the necessary changes, and still protect the individual's civil liberties, was the problem. The current law, that the person must present an "imminent danger" to self or others, was changed to allow involuntary treatment if it can be shown that "the person will, in the near future, cause serious physical harm to himself or others as evidenced by recent behavior causing, attempting, or threatening harm." TAC, and countless others, believed that the legislators fell short, leaving Virginia with one of the most restrictive laws for involuntary commitment in the nation.

The Treatment Advocacy Center would have preferred that Virginia model its involuntarily commitment law after one closer to Idaho's: that the person has an inability to provide for "any of his basic needs for nourishment, or essential medical care, or shelter or safety." Or the recent Illinois legislation that became state law on June 2008: "...because of the nature of his or her illness, is unable to understand his or her need for treatment and who, if not treated, is at risk of suffering or continuing to suffer mental deterioration or emotional deterioration, or both, to the point that the person is at risk of engaging in dangerous conduct." "Dangerous conduct" is defined as "threatening behavior or conduct that places another individual in reasonable expectation of being harmed, or a person's inability to provide, without the assistance of family or outside help, for his or her basic physical needs so as to guard himself or herself from serious harm." Thanks to the Illinois legislature, a person such as Seung Hui Cho can now be treated before a single shot spills blood on a classroom floor.

Under Illinois law, Cho would have been involuntarily committed to a mental hospital, and treated with a combination of pharmacology and psychotherapy, and housed in a controlled environment. He would have been released when, and if, the symptoms of his mental disorder were reduced to an acceptable level. We can only speculate as to the extent of Cho's potential recovery; for the unfortunate few whose brain is broken beyond repair, pills and therapy and prayers might not ever be enough.

Receiving proper care in a mental hospital is the first step in preparing patients for the outside world. What happens after they are released becomes the community's concern. Each time Becca was discharged the healing process stalled. The daily regime of medications soon came to an end. "I handled the abuse better when I was off my meds," Becca once said. "I could deal with anything when I was manic." The psychotherapy ended as well, and her environment, with all of its physical and sexual abuse, was worse than one could imagine. Clearly her only hope was to take the initiative to make certain that she continued her medication and her psychotherapy, and sought out a site where she could heal. But to negotiate the maze of mental health services required a clear-headed person, not someone who was actively mentally ill. The irony of the system is that one needs to be sane in order to find help for her insanity.

Larry L Franklin

No Need for a Prison Cell

It happened on a chilly April evening in the early 1970's, wrote Mary Ann Test, a psychologist in the School of Social Work at the University of Wisconsin-Madison. She loves to tell the story about how a group of impassioned mental health activists changed the way the nation, and perhaps the world, view mental health treatment for people who suffer from a serious mental illness. At the time, Test was the associate director and Arnold Marx, MD was the director of a research unit at the Mendota State Hospital in Madison. On that April evening, so the story goes, Mary Ann Test and Arnold Marx chaired a semi-annual staff meeting to evaluate the performance of recently discharged patients who suffered from schizophrenia, and to devise new and better ways of preparing them for their transition into the community. They met, as they had often done, in Building 2 (B-2), an aged one-story, weatherboard structure next to the Mendota State Hospital. Rather than focus on the evening's agenda, they wondered out loud why the attendance was so low. Time after time the staff had watched the hard-earned gains from inpatient care quickly erode after a patient was discharged, and returned to the hospital in worse condition than before. All of the staff's planning and hard work seemed to be in vain. They were demoralized.

B-2 was about to become the incubator for the birth of a new treatment philosophy. Over the next four hours, staff members talked and yearned for a different approach that might help patients deal with the outside community. And then one paraprofessional said, "What about Barb Lontz?" Lontz was an innovative, high-energy social worker whose clients never returned to Mendota. Lontz had taken community treatment to a different level; she had expanded the meaning of mental health care. The services she provided to her clients read like a laundry list: She helped her clients with their discharge planning; drove them to their new residences; helped them move in, and even put sheets on the beds; had their telephones installed; taught them how to use the laundromat, and how to ride the bus to the mental health center to get their medications; gave clients and family members her telephone number and said to call her anytime of the day or night; and if an emergency arose, she drove to the site and intervened. And then someone in the group said, "You know, I think the community, not the hospital, is where our patients need the most help. They adjust to the hospital quite well but life out in the community is hard, and it's especially hard for them... We ought to close B-2 down and all go out into the community like Barb and help our clients our there, where they really need support and where it will do the most good."

Mary Ann Test, together with psychiatrists Arnold Marx and Leonard Stein, had recognized the problem as far back as the 1960s. As directors of the research unit at Mendota, they had observed the hard-earned gains from inpatient care evaporate after a patient was released. It was clear to them that round-the-clock care alleviated the patient's symptoms, and that continued care was needed after discharge. This time they listened, and were moved by the youthful exuberance of the staff from B-2. This time they dared to be bold. The experience of Test, Marx, and Stein, was integrated with the energized staff into a force that was about to change the philosophy of community mental health care for people throughout the state, and eventually, throughout the nation.

In 1972, Marx, Stein, and Test moved a team of hospital staff into the community, launching a treatment model which would become known as Assertive Community Treatment (ACT). Unlike more traditional community-based treatment, ACT was developed for people with severe mental illness. The traditional model is a linkage or brokerage case-management program that connects the patient with a host of mental health, housing, or rehabilitation agencies in the community where the patient is treated by a group of individual case managers, each responsible for his own caseloads. The ACT model, based on a multi-disciplinary staff trained in the areas of psychiatry, social work, nursing, substance abuse, and vocational rehabilitation, works in a collaborative effort to deliver treatment, rehabilitation, and support services. The patient becomes a client of the entire staff. The days of working their way through the maze of community mental health services were over. They would, instead, be led by a team of committed advocates dedicated to the well-being of each client.

A typical ACT team consists of ten to twelve professionals – a psychiatrist, case managers, nurses and social workers, vocational specialists and peer specialists as well – who provide round-the-clock service, 7 days a week, 365 days a year. Each team member – trained in the areas of psychiatry, social work, nursing, substance abuse, and vocational rehabilitation – is capable of intervening with a client at any time. The team meets daily to discuss the clients assigned to their unit, and then determine what, if any, adjustments need to be made. While flexibility, a key ingredient of the team approach, allows them to design an individualized treatment plan dependent upon the severity of the mental illness, compassion, a sometimes overlooked component, raises mental health care to a more intimate level, giving clients the respect they had seldom experienced before.

***

It was 2003, the year that America invaded Iraq, and some 250,000 mentally ill walked our city streets or were caged like chickens in a city jail. Although $10 billion dollars were being spent on the war each month, we somehow lacked the money to treat the mentally ill. The lone bright spot was the growing acceptance of the Assertive Community Treatment programs of the 1970's that had become an established treatment model throughout communities across the nation. Three decades after the work of Mary Ann Test and her co-workers in building B-2, Karen Ring brought a new dimension to the model. She became the first "recovery specialist" in the state of Indiana, and perhaps in the nation, to be added to the ACT team. (A recovery specialist is a person who has advanced in their own recovery from a severe mental disorder, and is working to assist other people with a similar illness.) Karen treats the sickest of the sick, those with schizophrenia, bipolar disorder, clinical depression, or some form of psychosis. Her clients come from everywhere – some in family homes, maybe an apartment, a shelter home, hospitals, and the back streets and alleys of Indianapolis.

Karen's mental illness surfaced in 1972 when she was barely seventeen, a time of life when she might have gone to college, planned her future, and just enjoyed being young. But something happened in her brain. Maybe a few neurons twisted, turned, and shorted out; maybe the neurotransmitters fired blanks; or perhaps it was simply a genetic flaw in an otherwise beautiful mind. She was first diagnosed with schizophrenia, and later that diagnosis was changed to bipolar disorder. She spent eight years in and out of mental hospitals. Three weeks in a private hospital were followed by several short-term stays, and finally, when the insurance ran out, eleven months in a state mental hospital. Memories of her confinements, particularly those in the quiet room, still weigh hard.

"What is a quiet room?" I asked as we talked over the telephone that night.

"That's where they put me when I was going mad," she answered. "It was a room without windows. A small glass plate was in the door so the orderlies could look in. And the light switch was outside the room. It was pitch dark." Her voice cracked and she swallowed hard as if to push a memory back into her imaginary lock box. "They strapped me down on a bed covered by a thin mattress and leather straps. If that didn't quiet me, they gave me a shot of Thorazine. It still haunts me."

A thirty-six year struggle with bipolar disorder gives Karen a hands-on expertise that professional training cannot replicate. She knows how far clients can fall before reaching bottom, the strength of the currents, the floating debris just around the bend, and the depth of the river that they must cross. As some might say; "She's one of us."

It was obvious in my conversations with Karen that she had found her calling. "This is my life," she said. "This is what I was meant to do." Karen went on to explain how she became a recovery specialist. It was May of 2003, she recalled. She was doing volunteer work – answering the telephone and clerical duties – for an Indiana chapter of the National Alliance on Mental Illness. With the ending of her nineteen year marriage and the everyday stress of a severe mental illness, it was a particularly difficult period in her life. She could have stopped taking her medications, or possibly have given in to the seduction of her depression and ended it all. Those are the temptations that continually confront people who suffer from a severe mental illness.

Karen's determination to control her illness impressed the staff at NAMI. So much so, that a couple of them suggested that Karen apply for a job that was about to open at the Adult and Child Community Treatment Center. The Center had received a grant which allowed for the creation of a new position, a recovery specialist. It was the premise of the grant that a person in control of a severe mental illness would be a valuable addition to an ACT staff. Karen was hired, and has recently completed her sixth year with the Center. Indiana has added six more recovery specialists over the past six years.

Over the thirty-six years since the ACT model was conceived in that aged, one-story structure called B-2, countless studies have documented its success: less hospital time, increased employment, higher earned income, more independent living, better social relationships and quality of life, and a reduction in the symptoms brought on by mental illness. In one such study, eighteen percent of the ACT clients were hospitalized during the first year; eighty-nine percent of the non-ACT treatment group were hospitalized over the same period. While the initial costs are somewhat higher than the more traditional community treatment methods, a lower cost ratio results when you add increased periods of hospitalization for patients treated by non-ACT programs. And the societal costs – suicide, incarceration, homelessness, and violent crimes – spread across our nation, like ripples through water, an incalculable cost by any measure.

The ACT model has evolved over the past three decades, and is sometimes modified to serve a unique population. Some centers augment the basic model with dialectical behavior therapy to better serve clients with borderline personality and related disorders. Others consider a step-down ACT program that adopts a "tiered" case management system, where different levels of treatment are structured to fit a client's needs.

The model – expanded by specialists in criminal justice – is sometimes used to prepare some mentally ill offenders for release into the community, and even as an alternative to incarceration. When working with the criminal population, ACT has the added responsibility of balancing individual rights, the need for treatment, and public safety. The level of violence among some severally mentally ill offenders is of public concern. Society has no tolerance for a violent inmate being released into the community; nor do they embrace community treatment as an alternative for incarceration. Thus, the need for a closely monitored working relationship between the criminal justice and mental health systems. Together they educate offenders on their criminal offense, mental illness and its ramifications, and the need to adhere to a medication regime and continuous mental health care.

Critics of ACT, and there are a few, believe that the model does little to promote long-lasting behavioral changes. They maintain that the clients are coerced into following prescribed conduct, and are sometimes "bullied" into making certain choices. These actions, they claim, infringe upon the individual rights of clients. While their criticisms are noteworthy, such problems most likely occur when staff, or a particular staff member, lacks the compassion and empathy needed to work with such a population.

"On paper it's perfect," Karen said, when I asked for her

thoughts on the ACT model. "But in reality, it still has some problems." Karen went on to explain that the model has limitations – we can't make clients take their medications or follow our recommendations. As long as the client is not a threat to themselves or another party, they cannot be involuntarily hospitalized or forced to follow treatment.

"The turnover in staff is another problem," Karen added. "In the past six years, only two of the original staff are still members of the team." The lack of continuity tends to disrupt the team's flow, and for the client, it's like getting a new therapist each year.

"If I can gain their trust, and they believe that I care, I have a chance in reaching them." Although most of Karen's clients have progressed in their recovery, she has lost two clients over the past six years.

"What happened to them?" I asked.

"They overdosed," she said.

"You mean they committed suicide?"

"I don't know. I just know that they took too many pills. It tears me up," she said, as her voice dropped off. "The staff say that I am too vested with my clients. But I can't help it. This is who I am, this is what I do."

In 2006, and again in 2009, the National Alliance on Mental Illness released its report card, "Grading the States." In both reports on the nation's mental health field, the average for all states remained unchanged – a grade of D. Six states received Bs, eighteen Cs, twenty-one Ds, and six Fs. The report was based on sixty-five criteria with four sub-categories – consumer and family empowerment, health promotion and measurement, financing and core treatment/recovery services, and community integration and social inclusion. Becca's home state of Illinois received a D, and led the nation in the number of people with a serious mental illness that were being warehoused in nursing homes. Indiana received a D as well. Michael J. Fitzpatrick, executive director of NAMI, said, "Mental health care in America is in a crisis... Too many people living with mental illness end up hospitalized, on the street, in jail or dead."

The ACT model represents hope in a maze of mental health services. The model is highly structured, and parallels the general premise that recovery is based on the need for medication, individual support/psychotherapy, and a controlled environment. Without the more disciplined approach, people who suffer from a severe mental illness have no safety net to catch them on their downward fall. They are left to float in the abyss of madness.

Our nation lacks the financial and moral commitment to apply what we already know. When we look at Seung Hui Cho, Andre Yates, Rebecca Bivens, and the countless others who grab our attention for the length of a news cycle, we have fallen short. It could be said that how a nation treats its mentally ill is a measure of the country's moral evolution; so much to see if we care to look, so much to experience if we could only feel. There can be little doubt that with proper mental health treatment, Becca would have traveled down a far different path. There would be no need for a prison cell. And Dani Bivens would not be dead.

Cherry Blossoms & Barren Plains

Epilogue

Winter Day, 2009

When an adult kills a child, another star is plucked from the sky. The sadness is deep and lasting, a horrific crime by any measure, and possibly the ultimate sin. The circumstances surrounding the act – was she mentally ill – is of little concern. Society leaps to the defense of a victim so young, and demands revenge. "Lock the killer away," they say, "and better yet, give her the death penalty." In time, the perpetrator becomes the unseen, perhaps a modern day leper, and ultimately, the forgotten.

The fear that someone might escape prosecution under the guise of mental illness has pushed legislators to write laws that make it virtually impossible for a defendant to use the insanity defense. Society has little empathy for a mentally ill person who commits a violent crime. They refuse to acknowledge the fact that free will is sometimes gone, and that accountability is not etched in stone. Modern science tells us that someone who suffers from a severe mental illness can sometimes kill and not be conscious of their actions. Their reality is distorted, confused, and downright crazy. I've heard it so many times from people who are bipolar: *When I was in a manic state, I didn't know what I was doing, and days later, I didn't remember what I had done.* Except for the grace of God, and the absence of a genetic flaw, we might have done the same.

Becca and I have completed a four year journey where we were overcome by sadness, savored the more tender moments, laughed a bit, and shared some secrets which will never be told. I now see Becca as a wonderful person who was overwhelmed by a mental illness that drove her to madness. The one who committed the unthinkable is now my friend.

I saw her world of Cherry Blossoms and Barren Plains, the pure beauty of cherry blossoms dipped in white, emblazoned with a touch of pink, rapturous and addictive, and co-inhabited by bails of hell blowing across barren plains. This mood disorder of shifting extremes swallowed her whole, into a world where madness distorted the landscape, and reality sometimes recorded no memories or recollections of what just passed her by.

For ten years now, Becca has lived in a gray-colored world,

somewhere between the Cherry Blossoms and Barren Plains, in a prison called the Dwight Correctional Center. It's neither heaven nor hell; it's purgatory. Some inmates see purgatory as a place in between, a limbo of sorts, or possibly a physical or mental state of everlasting torment. Others believe it to be a temporary place, where the soul is cleansed and rehabilitated before ascending to the outside world. Those who have been unjustly convicted, or who suffer from a severe mental illness, wonder why their lives seem to have no purpose. They look for a hint of logic that might enlighten them about why their path has brought them here. Most believe, or hope, that they are part of some grand plan, and that God has not forgotten them. Once they have endured the fire, they will surely ascend to heaven, where the streets are paved in gold, misery is not even a memory, and life is a state of grace and godliness.

Living in a prison is especially difficult for someone who is mentally ill. Stress, loneliness, and fear of violence do not allow wounds to heal. Losing contact with your family is devastating as well. For the first eight years of Becca's incarceration, she had weekly visits with her older daughter, who lives some thirty to forty minutes from the Dwight Correctional Center. But over the past two years, the visits have tapered off to a mere one time a year, or perhaps not at all. (Her daughter became a mother and now works full time.)

Carolyn, Becca's mother, who is now widowed, lives on the east coast with Becca's three younger children. Although Carolyn visits Becca two times a year, Carolyn has never allowed the children to see their mother. Becca is left with the occasional letter or photograph to relive a child's birthday, graduation, or maybe a ride on her first bicycle. It's a sadness that Becca can ill afford, and one that she refuses to discuss.

Although the pastor, Raymond Rickert – a righteous man by any measure – retired and moved to Arkansas, he still manages to return to the Dwight Correctional Center two or three times a year. I have seen Becca numerous times over the past four years, and maintained a connection with letters and telephone calls. But Pastor Rickert and I are not family.

Becca's family circled the wagons and refused to contribute to the telling of her story. Instead, their reaction has been one of outrage, followed by her mother's threat to never speak to her again. I can only wonder what their reasons might be. Maybe they are embarrassed by the attention her story might bring; you don't let other people see your dirty laundry; the memories are too difficult to relive; Becca is where she belongs, enough said; or maybe they feel a level of guilt for not intervening on Becca's behalf before it was too late. Becca decided to tell her story so that others may learn about mental illness, in the hope that society will take a more active role in eliminating such preventable tragedies; and she wants her children to know the truth about their mother.

Short of an intervention from the Governor, Becca's only hope for a discharge is a reduction in her sentence to "time served." To date, her sentence has been reduced from a life sentence to forty years. With ten years completed, Becca has thirty more to serve. At an annual cost of $32,266., the State of Illinois has paid $322,660. for her first ten years of incarceration. Not counting inflation, and increases in the cost-of-living, they will pay an additional $979,800. for the completion of the next thirty years. That's a total cost of $1,302,460 to the State of Illinois. When do we say enough is enough? With proper treatment – and we do know that treatment works – Becca could become a contributing member of society in just a few years. She could become a tax paying citizen, and perhaps even strengthen the moral fiber of our nation. Is it worth spending an additional $979,800 for the sake of accountability, or maybe I should say revenge?

One day, not long ago, when Becca and I were sitting at a little round table in the visit room, I asked her what she thought that society should do with her.

"They should send me to a mental hospital for a few years and then let me go home," she said.

Being somewhat surprised by her response I asked, "Don't you think that they should let you out today?"

"No," she answered. "I'm not ready. I have some issues to work out. If I get the right help, I could be ready in a few years. Then they should let me go home."

LaVergne, TN USA
02 November 2010

203247LV00001B/7/P